7.95

M-Mode Echocardiographic Techniques and Pattern Recognition

M-Mode Echocardiographic Techniques and Pattern Recognition

SONIA CHANG

Assistant Professor of Medicine and Pediatrics
Medical College of Ohio at Toledo

Consultant, Riverside Hospital
Consultant, St. Vincent's Hospital
Toledo, Ohio

Lea & Febiger • *Philadelphia*

Library of Congress Cataloging in Publication Data

Chang, Sonia.
M-mode echocardiographic techniques and pattern recognition

Includes index.
1. Ultrasonic cardiography. I. Title.
[DNLM: 1. Echocardiography. WG141 C456m]
RC683.5.U5C48 616.1'2'0754 75-33110
ISBN 0-8121-0555-9

Published in Great Britain by Henry Kimpton Publishers, London

Printed in the United States of America

Print number 4 3 2

to

the cardiac patient

FOREWORD

Echocardiography, particularly its techniques and interpretation, is a topic that is commonly given only brief mention or omitted entirely from most medical publications. In this monograph, an invaluable addition to the literature, Sonia Chang describes the specific details of performing the echocardiographic examination, as well as some of the "tricks of the trade" which she has learned during her career in this field.

Although no one can become an expert in echocardiography by merely reading a text, one can become better informed and thus more proficient. The end result, of course, should be an increase in the number of patients who will benefit from this examination. Since the echocardiographer must be able to recognize both normal and abnormal tracings, illustrations of both are provided.

I am proud to have been Sonia Chang's mentor and honored to have been asked to write this foreword. Sonia Chang has made several important contributions to echocardiography. First, she has demonstrated that echocardiographic examinations do not have to be performed by physicians, and perhaps are better performed by people especially trained in these techniques. Because a quality echocardiographic tracing is the primary, and often sole, responsibility of the echocardiographic technologist, this person is certain to aim for the highest possible quality; an excellent tracing is a source of pride and satisfaction.

Another of Sonia Chang's contributions is the introduction of technical standards and innovations to the echocardiographic examination. Her constant emphasis on detail and quality has set standards for the world and has done much to advance the clinical usefulness of this technique. She has helped to develop and perfect a variety of new echocardiographic techniques, such as the M-mode scan, the condensed M-mode scan, and the subxiphoid examination.

Indeed, those who have learned echocardiography under my tutelage at Indiana University School of Medicine owe their high technical standards to Sonia Chang.

HARVEY FEIGENBAUM, M.D.

PREFACE

This procedure manual grew out of the need for an instructional source for the technical aspects of training visiting physicians and fellows rotating through the echocardiographic service at Indiana University, Indianapolis, Indiana, and at Emory University, Atlanta, Georgia.

The manual does not purport to be an atlas representative of all the pattern motions possible with the many cardiac lesions. It *does* attempt to give a ready and comprehensive reference to the physician and technician of the technical aspects of M-mode echocardiographic examination and possible pitfalls in recording and interpreting the more common cardiac abnormalities by this noninvasive procedure.

The illustrations are the results of studies conducted on equipment described in the publications from the Indiana University Echocardiographic Laboratory. However, the techniques used to obtain the illustrations are applicable to almost any type of commercially available equipment designed for echocardiography. Usually only minor modification of equipment is needed to duplicate the tracings described herein.

Most of these tracings were taken from adults with normal anatomical relationship of the intracardiac structures. Complex congenital anomalies are basically worked out using the techniques described in this manual. The interested reader should refer to the literature for more detailed descriptions of the manifestations of complex congenital disease as defined with M-mode echocardiography.

SONIA CHANG

ACKNOWLEDGMENTS

I have just come through eight of the most intellectually exciting years of my life. Contributing to the content of those years have been leaders in echocardiography, hospital staff members, visiting physicians, technicians, engineers and patients. From publications and lectures of other investigators, from friendly discussions and from heated arguments have come seeds of ideas leading to the development of an established protocol for routine M-mode echocardiographic examination.

Several people have played major roles in my development as an echocardiographer at Indiana University from 1967 to 1975. To them I express my deepest gratitude and thanks for their instruction, guidance, moral support and daily assistance. To:

Richard Campbell, M.D., who first guided me through the intricacies of intracardiac hemodynamics;

John Chang, my husband, who conceived the idea and encouraged the growth of this procedure manual throughout the years when physicians came to this laboratory for echocardiographic instruction;

James Dillon, M.D., whose sense of humor was always appreciated;

Harvey Feigenbaum, M.D., a highly imaginative and innovative employer, mentor and friend, who encouraged me to leave the cardiac catheterization laboratory and take up echocardiography at a time when this diagnostic procedure was still in its infancy;

Raymond Gramiak, M.D., Michael Johnson, M.D., and Claude Joyner, M.D., from whom I borrowed and modified techniques for examining the aortic valve and great vessels, prosthetic Starr-Edwards valves and the mitral valve, respectively;

Janie Stewart, a superb technician and friend, without whom I would never have had the time to put this manual together in its present format had she not assumed the tedious details that keep a very busy laboratory functioning smoothly;

Arthur (Ned) Weyman, M.D., friend and colleague, contributor par excellence to the field of echocardiography;

Phil Wilson, for his illustrative ability with pen, ink and paint brush; for instruction in how to turn an ordinary tracing into a work of art;

And, finally, to Joe Demma, Carol Eitzen, Donald Izban and Donald Schoch who patiently mounted and printed innumerable illustrations.

SONIA CHANG

CONTENTS

1

INTRODUCTION

Echocardiography and the Physician

Since the physician is responsible for the interpretation and disposition of an echocardiographic reading, it is necessary for him to become an expert in the complexities of the examination before attempting to teach technicians. There is no way for the physician to circumvent the need to be knowledgeable and adept in the application of this method to diagnose cardiac disease.

So far the responsibility for training echocardiographic technicians has fallen to individual physicians who employ them. The advantages in this relationship are numerous: The physician is available to answer questions, describe a disease or correct technique on a daily basis over a long interval. No short-term courses for the technician can substitute for this teaching-learning situation. Both physician and technician benefit from this type of interaction. In a close working relationship the physician can reinforce his own confidence that technically satisfactory examinations are being obtained. Through medical meetings and current literature the physician can keep abreast of advances in the field and apply this information in his own laboratory.

Echocardiography and the Technician

Echocardiography has become a new career area, professionally recognized, for men and women who wish to have an active and intelligent role in the definitive diagnosis of the diseased heart. To date the most readily available source of potential echocardiographers consists of personnel from the field of nursing and from catheterization and phonocardiographic laboratories. These workers can immediately utilize their background in cardiac anatomy and hemodynamics to record and interpret echocardiographic tracings under proper supervision and long-term instruction by the physician. However, any person with a lively curiosity, bold imagination, willingness to learn and considerable patience has the potential to become an efficient echocardiographer. Manual dexterity has become an important factor. Some artistic inclinations, including an appreciation for the beauty of a well-done echogram, are necessary ingredients for a competent echocardiographer.

The echocardiographic examination is unlike any other type of ultrasound procedure. Because the heart is a dynamic organ, reflecting the hemodynamics within its chambers, the art of recording meaningful tracings must be acquired at the bedside. Classroom teaching is useful to educate the examiner about diseases that may be identified by echocardiography. Patterns of motion to be expected from specific cardiac disease can be learned and by comparing tracings from many sources, one can follow the "state of the art." But only by having the transducer in one's hand and examining several hundred patients personally, can one achieve expertise in recording echocardiographic tracings.

Technicians should utilize ancillary activities to aid their "basic education" at the bedside. Attendance at conferences is useful. At such meetings patients are presented who have been studied with electrocardiography, echocardiography, phonocardiography, treadmill exercises and cardiac catheterization. At this time diagnostic studies and further medical management of the patient are discussed; the technician may see the overall picture of the patient's clinical status and treatment. This personalization of every examination keeps echocardiography from becoming just another static diagnostic procedure.

Generalized reading on the most common types of acquired heart disease and of common congenital disease is also helpful. Particular attention to the anatomical structure of the normal and congenitally deformed hearts is essential. Short, in-depth discussions of cardiac abnormalities and hemodynamics with staff members who are willing to teach are invaluable.

There is no shortcut to becoming a proficient echocardiographer. Efforts to help educate the technician have been persistently attempted through organized courses, regional meetings and short-term visits to other laboratories. All these efforts and others are needed, but all experienced echocardiographers agree that the most useful teaching-learning process lies in the harmonious cooperation between the echocardiographic physician and his technician in their own laboratory.

Suggested Reading

Baum, G.: Application of ultrasound. JAMA, *229*:1065, 1974.

Belenkie, I.: Echocardiography. J. Med. Assoc. Ga., *61*:143, 1972.

Bender, F., *et al.*: Diagnosis of primary tumors of the heart. Minerva Med., *64*:1692, 1973.

Child, J., Abbasi, A., and Pearce, M: Echocardiographic differentiation of mediastinal tumors from primary cardiac disease. Chest, *67*:108, 1975.

Cooper, R., and Leopold, G.: Diagnostic ultrasound in cardiology. Med. Ann. DC, *41*:748, 1972.

Cortina, A., and Lopez-Bescos, L.: Ultrasonics in cardiology. Rev. Esp. Cardiol., *26*:15, 1973.

Dillon, J., and Feigenbaum, H.: Echocardiography, 1974. J. Indiana State Med. Assoc., *67*:104, 1974.

Effert, S.: Ultrasonic diagnosis of heart disease. Fortschr. Geb. Roentgenstr. Nuklearmed., Suppl. *24*:1972.

Feigenbaum, H.: Spotting disease by ultrasound. Cardiovascular Review. Medical World News, 1970.

Feigenbaum, H.: Clinical applications of echocardiography. Prog. Cardiovasc. Dis., *14*:531, 1972.

Feigenbaum, H.: Echocardiography. Philadelphia, Lea & Febiger, 1972.

Feigenbaum, H.: Echocardiography. Cardiovascular Review. World Medical News, 1973.

Feigenbaum, H.: Newer aspects of echocardiography. Circulation, *47*:833, 1973.

Feigenbaum, H.: Ultrasound as a clinical tool in valvular heart disease. Cardiovasc. Clinics, Valvular Heart Disease (Vol. 5). No. 2, p. 219, Philadelphia, F. A. Davis, 1973.

Feigenbaum, H.: Educational problems in echocardiography. Am. J. Cardiol., *34*:741, 1974 (editorial).

Feigenbaum, H.: Hazards of echocardiographic interpretation. N. Engl. J. Med., *289*:1311, 1974 (editorial).

Feigenbaum, H., Dillon, J., and Chang, S.: Recent developments in echocardiography. *In* New Horizons in Cardiovascular Practice, Edited by H. I. Russek. Baltimore, University Park Press, p. 75, 1975.

Freyler, H.: Urgent ultrasonic echocardiography. Klin. Monatsbl. Augenheilkd., *162*:373, 1973.

Goldberg, S., Allen, H., and Sahn, D.: Pediatric and Adolescent Echocardiography: A Handbook. Chicago, Yearbook Medical, 1975.

Goldschoager, S., *et al.*: Right atrial myxoma with right to left shunt and polycythemia presenting as congenital heart disease. Am. J. Cardiol., *30*:82, 1972.

Gramiak, R.: Cardiac ultrasonography. A review of current applications. Radiol. Clin. North Am., *9*:469, 1971.

Gramiak, R.: Echocardiography. JAMA, *229*:1099, 1974.

Gramiak, R., *et al.*: Report of the inter-society commission for heart disease resources. Optimal resources for ultrasonic examination of the heart. J. Clin. Ultrasound *3*:2, 1975.

Harbold, N., Jr., and Gau, G.: Echocardiographic diagnosis of right atrial myxoma. Mayo Clin. Proc., *48*:284, 1973.

Holmes, J.: Diagnostic Ultrasound (3 Vols). The office of Post-Graduate Medical Education, Container #C295. Denver; University of Colorado School of Medicine.

Joyner, C.: Echocardiography. Circulation *46*:835, 1972 (editorial).

Joyner, C.: Ultrasound in the diagnosis of cardiovascular pulmonary disease. Chicago, Yearbook Medical, 1974.

Kerber, R.: Errors in performance and interpretation of echocardiograms. J. Clin. Ultrasound, *1*:330, 1973.

King, J., Gray, W., and Dunn, M.: Echocardiography. Clinical applications of echocardiography. J. Kans. Med. Soc., *73*:284, 1972.

Lele, P. P.: Application of ultrasound in medicine. N. Engl. J. Med., *286*:1317, 1972.

McDicken, W. N.: Annual meeting of the BMUG on clinical applications of diagnostic ultrasound. Ultrasonics, *11*:137, 1973.

Mason, D.: Non-invasive cardiology, a new horizon. Calif. Med., *119*:53, 1973.
Mason, D.: Non-invasive methods for the assessment of cardiac function. Calif. Med., *119*:21, 1973.
Mukharliamov, N., and Belenkov, I.: Use of echocardiography in diagnosis of the diseases of the cardiovascular system. Ter. Arkh., *46*:3, 1974.
Nimura, Y.: A primer to echocardiogram (author's translation). Respir. Circ. (Tokyo), *21*:1051, 1973.
Pernod, J.: Indications of ultrasonic echography in cardiology. J. Radiol. Electrol. Med. Nucl., *53*:701, 1972.
Popp, R., and Harrison, D.: Echocardiography in non-invasive cardiology. Edited by A. M. Weissler. New York, Grune and Stratton, p. 149, 1974.
Ross, F.: Ultrasonic investigation of heart. *In* Ultrasonics in Clinical Diagnosis. Edited by P. Wells. Edinburgh and London, Churchill Livingstone, p. 120, 1972.
Rost, R., and Schneider, K. W.: Possibilities in the use of echocardiography. Fortschr. Med., *92*:3, 1974.
Rost, R., and Schneider, K. W.: Possibilities in the use of echocardiography. Conclusion. Fortschr. Med., *92*:65, 1974.
Schneider, K. W., *et al.*: Comparison of heart catheterization and ultrasonic cardiogram findings. Radiologe, *12*:137, 1972.
Schneider, K. W., *et al.*: Comparative study on the results of heart catheterization and echocardiography. Fortschr. Geb. Roentgenstr. Nuklearmed. Suppl. 24, 1972.
Segel, E., *et al.*: Echocardiography. Current concepts and clinical application. Am. J. Med., *57*:267, 1974.
Stefan, G.: Echocardiography: Clinical Use—Advantages—Limitations (author's translation). Munch. Med. Wochenschr., *116*(13):659, 1974.
Stefan, G.: Echocardiography. Value—Advantages—Limitations. Minerva Med., *65*:2887, 1974.
Tanaka, M., *et al.*: Ultrasonic evaluation of anatomical abnormalities of heart in congenital and acquired heart disease. Br. Heart J., *33*:686, 1971.
Venco, A., Finardi, G., and Saviotti, M.: Evaluation of some internal dimensions of the heart and great vessels by echocardiography (author's translation). G. Ital. Cardiol., *4*:173, 1974.
Walter, J., Ruh, P., and Dale, G.: Echography in cardiology. J. Radiol. Electrol. Med. Nucl., *53*:705, 1972.

2

INSTRUMENTATION

All the techniques in this manual can be adapted to echographic instruments with strip chart recorders. Practically none of the scanning techniques can be recorded on Polaroid camera apparatus, although the techniques are used to visually locate one structure in relation to another. The condensed scan techniques require strip chart recorders with recording capabilities of 10 mm/sec and superb resolution. However, any scan may be recorded at faster speeds, and the dimensions measured as desired.

Good housekeeping of the equipment is essential for optimal operation and trouble-free years of use. Be sure to:

1. Keep air filters clean.
2. Wipe transducers off after each examination to prevent corrosion of the facing material.
3. Check the focusing of the echograph and strip chart recorder periodically, especially if many portable studies are done. The jiggling over elevator door bases and uneven tunnels may disturb the focusing. Also, if many people use the echograph, someone invariably turns the wrong knob.
4. Check electrocardiogram leads periodically for wear or breakage.
5. Damp-mop the coupling gel from the equipment to prevent corrosion and staining of cabinet and metals.
6. Keep a supply of slow-blow fuses on hand.
7. Repair or replace worn-out or defective parts at the first sign of difficulty.

The first place to check when the echograph or strip chart recorder malfunctions is the numerous *fuses* on both instruments. Replacement of burned-out fuses will usually solve the problem, but only temporarily since there is an underlying cause for the trouble. Confer with service representatives. A simple adjustment or component replacement made promptly may save a large repair bill later.

Operating Controls

The description of the controls and their function in the instruction manuals accompanying the different types of echograph instruments is usually adequate. Most echographs have a set of controls that can be made to interact and produce very specific results in the graphic presentation of information from oscilloscope to paper or prints. These controls are commonly known as "reject," "near gain," "coarse gain," "damping" and "depth compensation." Although these controls are in different locations on different instruments, they all work in similar ways. Figure 1 shows the front panel of a commercially available echograph, which will serve as a representative model to facilitate discussion.

Reject

From the technician's point of view, reject is the control that eliminates low amplitude echoes from the system altogether. The

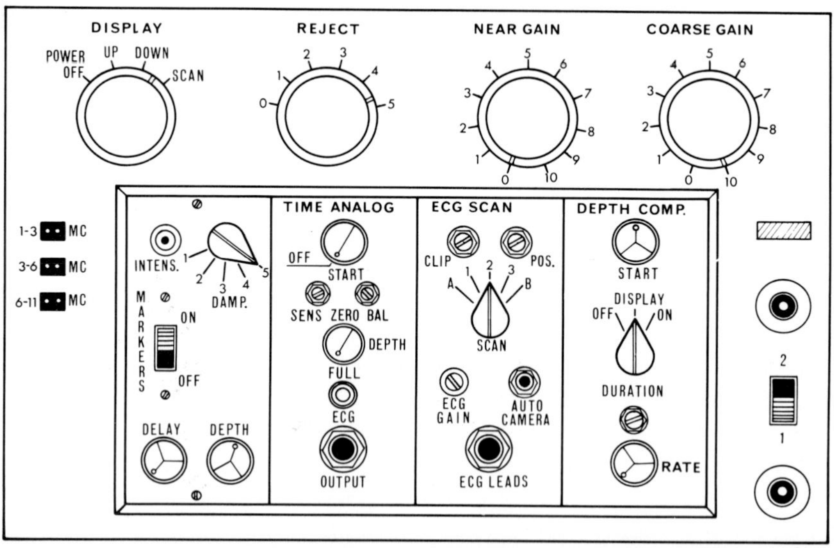

Figure 1. Front panel of commercially available echograph. Most tracings recorded in this manual used following settings: reject, 2 or 3; near gain, not more than 3; coarse gain, variable; damping, 3; depth compensation, maximum slope ending in midseptum.

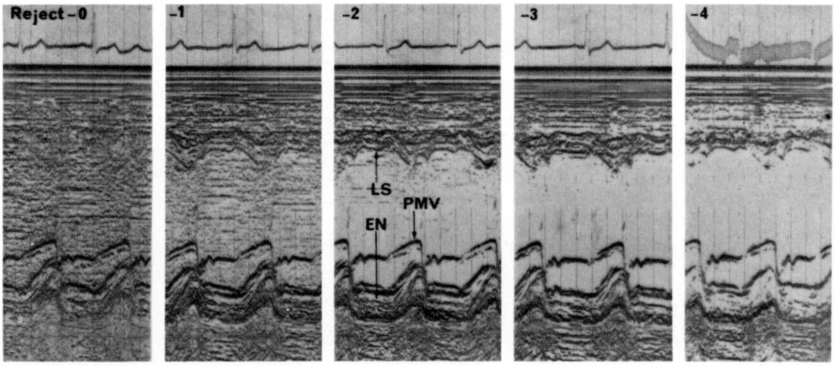

Figure 2. Effects of reject (see text). LS = left side of septum, EN = endocardial surface of posterior left ventricular wall and PMV = posterior mitral valve.

echoes no longer exist and cannot be acted on by gain or damping. If the reject is set on "0" or "1" (Figure 2), many echoes with very low amplitude are seen to fill the ventricular chamber between the left septum and the endocardium of the posterior left ventricular wall. These echoes do not contribute to the value of the study and are best eliminated by raising the reject to a higher level. The tracing in Figure 2 becomes more acceptable with the reject set on "2" or "3." All the structures that can be used for routine left ventricular measurements are clearly defined. By raising the reject to "4," too many echoes have been eliminated from the system and useful information is lost.

Gain

Gain is the control that amplifies echoes received from the transducer. It may be increased or decreased at will to make the recording graphically acceptable for measurements. Signals perpendicular to the structure being examined will be reflected as strong and solid lines on the tracing.

Gain will not improve the tracings if the transducer is incorrectly positioned on the patient's chest. Gain can only amplify those signals that are being received. It does *not* select those echoes which are most useful to make a diagnosis.

Near Gain

Near gain controls the amplitude of those echoes received from the transducer and which are located between the crystal artifact (Figure 3) and the depth compensation ramp (Figure 5).

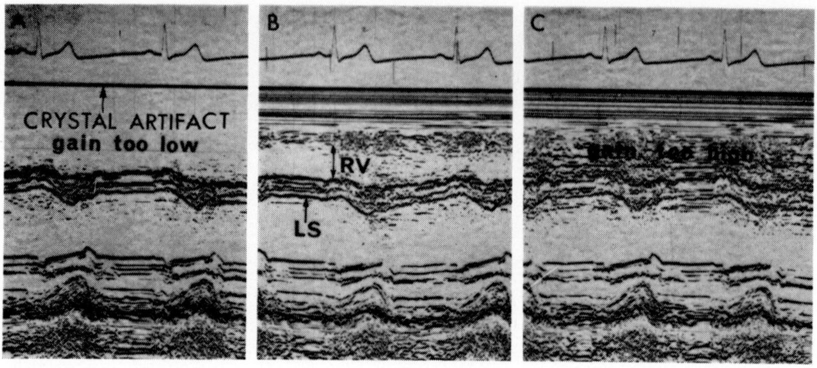

Figure 3. Effects of near gain when depth compensation ramp is ending at right side of septum. Near gain controls amplitude of those echoes received between crystal artifact and end of depth compensation ramp. *A*, Near gain was turned off; *B*, near gain is properly set at low level so that only structures which are useful are observed, in this case chest wall and right ventricular wall; *C*, near gain was turned too high. Useful structures cannot be identified at this level of amplification, and usefulness of "near gain" is defeated. RV = right ventricle and LS = left side of septum.

In Figure 3*A* the near gain has been turned completely off, so that no echoes are being received in the area between the crystal artifact and the right side of the septum. In Figure 3*B* the near gain has been increased to a level just high enough to amplify echoes from the chest wall, the right ventricular wall and anything else which may lie in the pathway of the sound beam between the right ventricular wall and the right side of the septum. Sometimes the tricuspid valve may be seen if the right ventricle is dilated. Figure 3*C* displays the effect of too much amplification of echoes being received between the crystal artifact and the right side of the septum. The right ventricular wall cannot be identified, and an accurate right ventricular dimension could not be taken.

Coarse Gain

Figure 4 demonstrates how coarse gain controls the amplitude of *all* received echoes equally. If the coarse gain is set too high, the dominant echoes such as the right and left sides of the septum will be poorly defined (Figure 4*B*). This is because echoes that are not essential to the quality of the study are being overamplified and thus seen and recorded with desired structures. If the coarse gain setting is too low, the septal and posterior left ventricular wall echoes appear broken and poorly defined (Figure 4*C*). The transducer is perpendicular to the septum and posterior left ventricular wall, but the coarse gain is too low to record the complete motion of these structures.

Figure 4*A* is the most acceptable tracing. The right and left side of

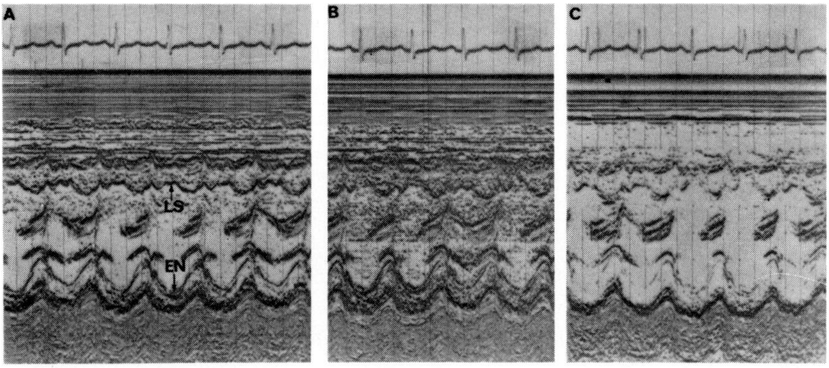

Figure 4. Effects of coarse gain (see text). *A,* Coarse gain set at suitable level to visualize motion of desired structures; *B*, coarse gain setting is too high, overamplifying desired structures; *C*, coarse gain setting is too low, causing some dropout of desired motion. LS = left septum and EN = endocardial surface of posterior left ventricular wall.

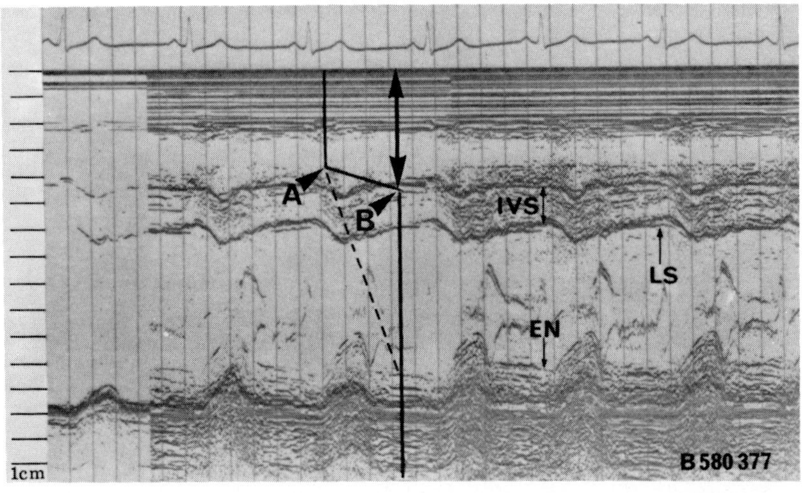

Figure 5. Depth compensation set so that ramp ends at right side of septum. Near gain controls amplification of echoes between crystal artifact and right side of septum (large arrow) without affecting amplification of signals received from left septum and endocardium of posterior left ventricular wall. *A*, Point at which received signals began to be amplified; *B*, point at which received signals achieve maximum amplification. Examiner may wish to compensate for strength of received signals more gradually, in which case ramp would have more gradual slope (dotted line). This accommodation is useful in patients with aortic insufficiency or coronary artery disease. IVS = interventricular septum, LS = left septum and EN = endocardial surface of posterior left ventricular wall.

the interventricular septum and the endocardial and pericardial surfaces of the posterior left ventricular wall are easily identified, and dimensions may be measured without difficulty. The near gain is set slightly too high. At a lower setting the right ventricular wall would be more clearly defined.

Depth Compensation

Without depth compensation any signal transmitted into soft tissue and received again would be strong near, and very weak in areas far away from, the transducer. Echoes received from the chest wall and right ventricular wall, for example, would be very strong; echoes received from the posterior left ventricular wall would be very weak. This is because the signal must pass through much tissue to reach the posterior wall; it must then be reflected back to the transducer. Along the way it is continually being absorbed or deflected by the tissue it passes through, becoming weaker and weaker. What is needed is one or more sets of controls that will suppress the strength of the signal near the transducer and amplify the far signals returning from the mitral valve and posterior left ventricular wall. Most echographs do in fact have these controls, which may be called "depth compensation" or "time-compensated gain."

I prefer to set the depth compensation in a position so that the maximum "ramp" *ends* at the right ventricular septum (Figure 5). Signals from the septum begin to be amplified at point A and reach maximum amplification at point B (Figure 5); the strength of the returning signals seems to be equalized from the right side of the septum to the endocardium thereafter. The "near gain" may then be adjusted so that the chest wall and right ventricular wall may be visualized without affecting the strength of the signals being returned from the septum and posterior wall.

The depth compensation must be adjusted to every individual patient so that the ramp *ends* at the right ventricular septum. If the ramp is too far forward toward the transducer, the near gain control cannot be used effectively; if the ramp is too far posterior, *i.e.*, behind the left septum or mitral valve, these structures may not be seen at all unless the near gain is increased to very high levels. Remember that near gain controls only those echoes lying between the crystal artifact and the depth compensation ramp, regardless of where the ramp is located.

Depth

Depth must be adjusted for every patient. This control is used to display variable amounts of tissue between the crystal artifact and the lung. If an examiner does a study on a patient with coronary artery disease with a very large heart, the depth will be compressed so that approximately 20 cm of tissue may be visualized. The next patient may be a small child. If the depth is not changed to accommodate the size of the child's heart, the tracing may be similar to that seen in Figure

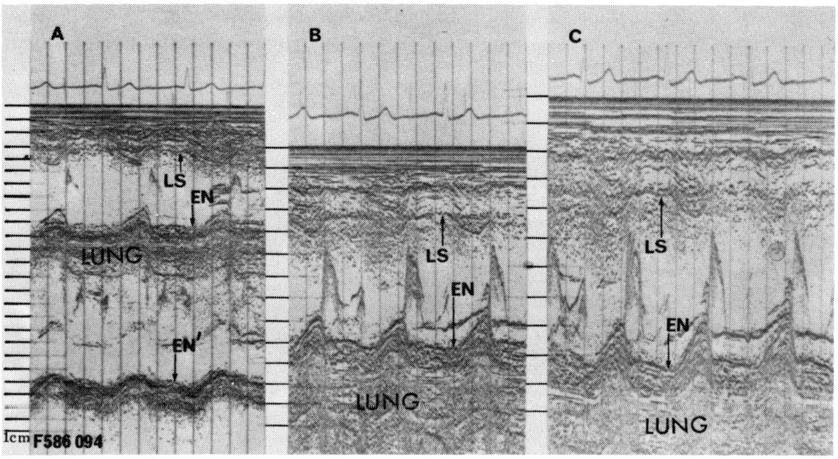

Figure 6. Effects of depth (see text). *A*, Tracing is compressed too much, allowing reverberations. Tracing should be expanded as in *B* so that most reverberations are eliminated from presentation; *C*, tracing has been expanded too much although interpretation is still relatively easy. Tracing on paper becomes light, and echoes, which may lie close together, are separated from each other and cause difficulty in determining which lines truly represent motion of structure desired. Although *C* does not illustrate this point, it should be kept in mind. Often there is a problem of deciding which lines represent true endocardium of posterior left ventricular wall. If tracing is more compressed, close-lying lines reinforce each other and appear as very strong signal. If tracing is excessively expanded, this reinforcing effect is lost. LS = left septum, EN = endocardial surface of posterior left ventricular wall and EN′ = reverberation from true endocardium.

6*A*. The desired left ventricular structures are in the top half of the tracing; the lower half of the tracing exhibits reverberations, which in too many cases have been misinterpreted.

An easy maneuver to follow from one patient to another is to set the depth scale at 15 cm, with the depth compensation ramp *ending* at 5 cm. If the heart is larger, the depth may be further compressed; if the heart is smaller, the depth may be expanded (Figure 6*B*). One can overexpand the depth, especially in children, and then the tracing becomes exceedingly difficult to interpret. After ventricular structures are identified, a rule of fourths should be followed, *i.e.*, one-fourth of the tracing for electrocardiogram and any other parameter desired; one-half of the paper width should be occupied by the echocardiogram; and one-fourth for lung, surprise pleural effusions or giant left atriums. For further discussion, refer to Figures 83 and 84.

Damping

Damping (or attenuation) controls the strength of the signal being *transmitted* from the transducer to the body. By increasing the damping

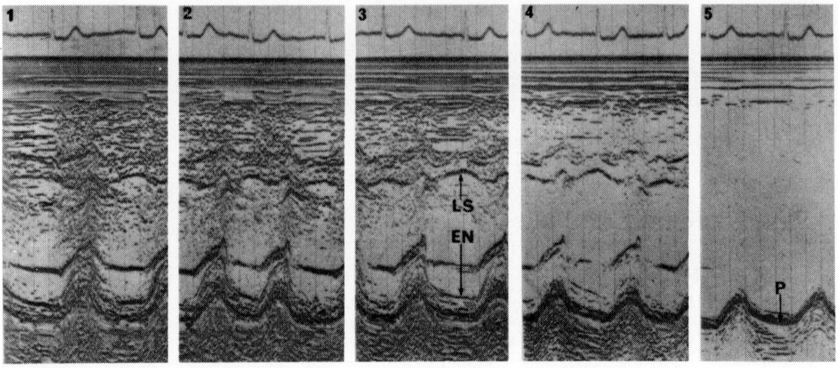

Figure 7. Effects of damping. *1,* Full-strength signal is being transmitted from transducer; unless coarse gain is decreased, there will be too many echoes in the tracing; *2* and *3*, damping progressively increased. Weaker signals are being transmitted, but quality of tracing is entirely acceptable; *4*, damping further increased. Some signals are too weak and cannot travel back to be received by transducer. Increasing coarse gain may amplify these echoes so that tracing is again acceptable; *5*, maximum damping has eliminated all echoes from system except pericardium which is strongest reflecting interface. LS = left septum, EN = endocardial surface of posterior left ventricular wall and P = pericardium.

(decreasing the strength of the signal transmitted), the examiner can effectively eliminate all echoes except the pericardial echo (Figure 7). By this method one can examine a heart for pericardial effusion. All echoes are eliminated from the system except close-lying echoes such as those from the pericardium and epicardium of the left ventricle. If there were any significant separation between these two structures, the presence of pericardial effusion could be identified (see p. 93 for discussion of pericardial effusion).

Transducers

Transducers come in many sizes, varying sensitivity, megaHertz range and focused or nonfocused. Depending on the patient population with which a laboratory is involved, a family of transducers should be acquired. Our laboratory has had success with transducers focused at 7.5 cm for adults or 5.0 cm for children. Currently we use nonfocused transducers with a test sensitivity of 39 decibels, 2.25 megaHertz and 0.5 inch diameter. For patients with very small intercostal spaces or for small children, we use transducers with 0.25-inch diameter, 2.25 or 3.25 megaHertz; for newborn infants, a 5.0 megaHertz transducer is utilized.

The megaHertz indicates the wavelength frequency, *i.e.*, the lower the megaHertz—1.6, *e.g.*—the longer the wavelength and therefore the greater the penetration into soft tissue. However, the resolution may not be very efficient. Resolution is defined as the ability to distinguish between close-lying echoes, as in pericardium-epicardium interfaces. Two separate echoes would be seen, rather than a single broad echo. This is considered to be good resolution. A frequency of 2.25-megaHertz seems to be adequate for most individuals from age 2 to 100 years. A transducer with a frequency of 3.25 or 5.0 megaHertz has a shorter wavelength, therefore less penetration, but the resolution is excellent. These are used on newborn babies, infants to age two years and in studies in which the exact thickness of the right ventricular wall is desired.

Coupling Gel

Coupling gel or jelly insures an air-free medium between the patient's skin and the transducer. One should consider those commercially available products which do not stain clothing, are hypoallergenic and will not melt at slightly elevated body temperatures.

If echograms are being taken at the bedside and the jelly is unavailable, substitutes with no adverse effects either to patient or to quality of the tracing include: hair cream, lubrifax, mineral oil, EKG paste, petrolatum, cold cream, hair setting gel (or similar product which the patient may have).

Mobile Carts for Echographic and Strip Chart Recording Equipment

If a laboratory has not already invested in equipment, the following considerations should be weighed when evaluating the purchase of equipment:

1. Will the equipment be laboratory based or will it make frequent trips to the intensive care units?
2. If the equipment is to be used as a portable system, can the technician push it farther than across the hall with minimum effort? (There is a big difference between movable and portable!)
3. Are the wheels of the cart sufficiently large to roll easily across elevator doorways without falling in the cracks?
4. Is there provision for storing an additional box of paper, coupling gel, tissues, transducers, small screwdriver, extra fuses, pencils and the completed tracing?
5. Is the echograph on the cart adjustable to the height of the examiner? Inability to adjust for height differences may cause strain for a particular examiner.

Polaroid Photographs

Many problems concerning the graphic appearance of an echocardiographic tracing taken on Polaroid film have nothing to do with the technical skill in obtaining the tracing. Basic adjustments must be made on the echograph that will optimize the focusing, intensity and

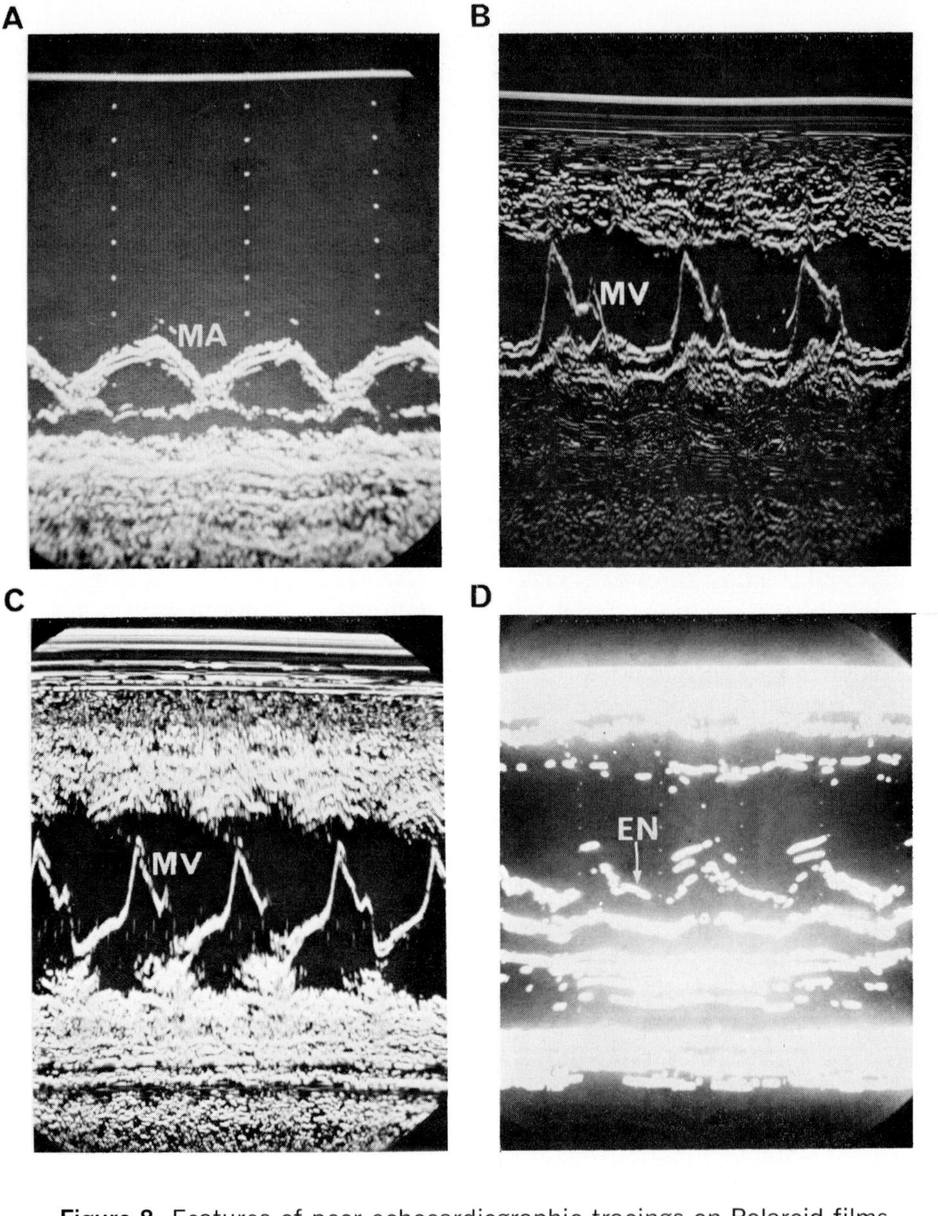

Figure 8. Features of poor echocardiographic tracings on Polaroid films. *A*, Intensity is too high. Mitral annulus was recorded with transducer positioned at apex and directed longitudinally through left ventricle; *B*, appearance of tracing when clipping is too low, or camera aperture size may be too small or intensity may be too low; *C*, tracing is out of focus; *D*, tracing exhibits "bloom." Clipping is set too high so that close-lying structures blend together, and resolution is reduced. MA = mitral annulus, MV = mitral valve and EN = endocardial surface of posterior left ventricular wall.

clipping. The interplay of these three controls affects the quality of the tracing on the film. Usually these adjustments are made and then remain stable, but if many persons use the echograph for different types of examination, then these control settings should be checked frequently.

Follow the recommendation in the echograph service manuals but also proceed as follows (Figure 8):

1. Panel C is out of focus. Focus the instrument with fine focus while the M-mode is sweeping or set on B-mode. Focus on the calibration dots until they are pinpoint. It is not necessary to do this very often unless a malfunction of the instrument causes the focusing to become unstable.
2. Panel A shows that the intensity is set too high. Place the damping (attenuation) on level 5 or turn the coarse gain all the way down. Adjust the intensity control until there is a faint band of light sweeping across the oscilloscope. If this adjustment is set too high, the whole photograph, including the background, will be too light and poorly defined.
3. Panel D demonstrates an effect called "bloom." The clip control is set too high. Apply jelly to the transducer and press against the palm of the hand. Place the damping on settings 1, 2 or 3, depending on the instrument. Set the near gain and coarse gain at moderate levels and the reject on 3, 4 or 5. Turn the CLIP completely clockwise, then turn it counterclockwise until every individual echo being received from the transducer can be distinguished.

   If the clip adjustment is too high as seen in panel D, echoes close to each other will bleed into large, fuzzy images with poor resolution.
4. Take a picture of the oscilloscope with echoes being displayed. If the picture is too dark as in panel B, turn the clip up slightly. Take another picture. If the oscilloscope display looks very good but the picture is still to dark, increase the size of the camera aperture to admit more light. A setting of *f*5.6 is usual but settings between *f*8 and *f*16 have been used by different examiners. If the picture seems overexposed, decrease the size of the camera aperture to admit less light.
5. Do not be concerned if calibration markers are not seen on the photographs. Quality tracings of the echocardiogram are desired first. Calibrations may be taken at the end of the examination on a separate photograph without any tracing.

3

MITRAL VALVE

An echocardiographic examination is begun by positioning the patient in a supine or partial left lateral position, the head and thorax being slightly elevated to about 30° (Figure 9).

Initially the transducer is placed along the left sternal border in the third or fourth intercostal space. From this position the mitral valve should be located. If it cannot be located, the transducer should be moved systematically over the precordium and shifted to higher or lower intercostal spaces until the mitral valve or aorta can be visualized. Just because one begins in the third intercostal space is no reason to have to stay there. Many patients have been monitored from the fifth and sixth intercostal spaces, and from others it has been impossible to obtain echoes through the chest. In these latter cases the subxiphoid examination is utilized (see p. 117).

The mitral valve is used as a reference point to locate all other cardiac structures (Figure 10). The pulmonary valve lies superior to the mitral valve in a plane with the left ear; the aortic valve lies in a sector between the throat and right shoulder; the tricuspid valve lies directly medial to the mitral valve; and last, the apex lies in an inferior and lateral plane below the mitral valve. Obviously a left ventricular study lies between the mitral valve and the apex.

Imagine the transducer as an extended ice pick. The smallest angle change of the transducer (A in Figure 11) causes a considerable angle change at the end of the ultrasonic beam (B in Figure 11). Most echocardiographers who have difficulty trying to record cardiac structures that are in close proximity angle the transducer too sharply and overshoot the structure that they are trying to record.

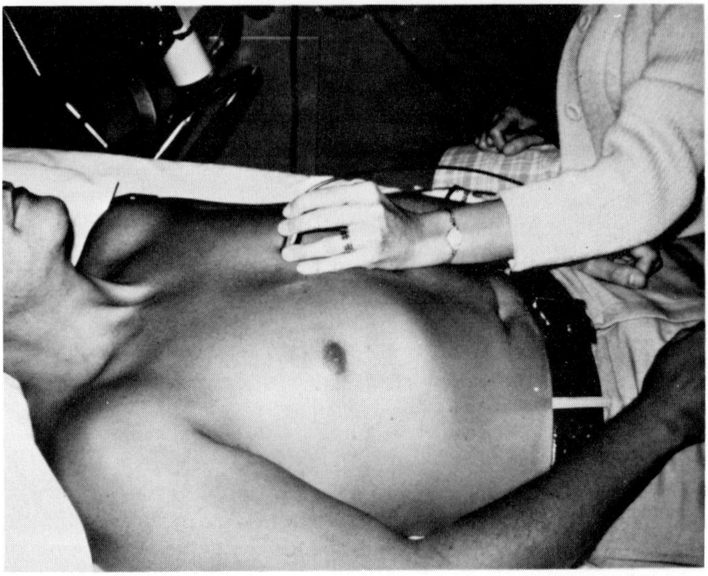

Figure 9. Interrelationship of patient, examiner and echographic equipment. Although examiner and equipment are positioned on left side of bed in illustration, examiner and equipment may as easily be positioned on right side of patient—transducer would then, of course, be held in examiner's right hand.

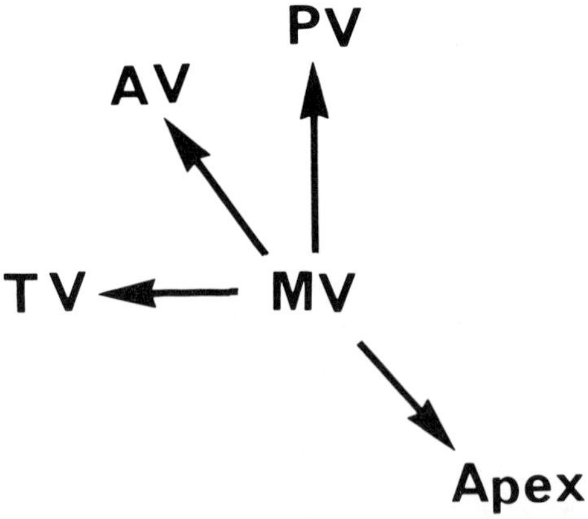

Figure 10. Interrelationship of cardiac valves and apex of left ventricle. MV=mitral valve, PV=pulmonary valve, AV=aortic valve and TV=tricuspid valve.

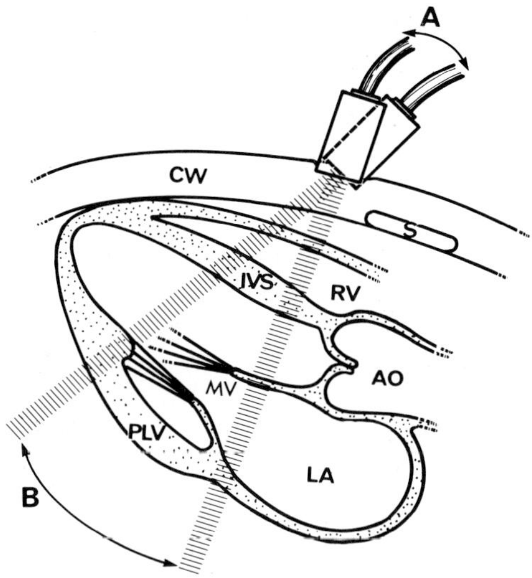

Figure 11. Position of ultrasound beam in relation to posterior wall as angle of transducer is changed. CW = chest wall, IVS = interventricular septum, RV = right ventricle, S = sternum, AO = aorta, LA = left atrium and PLV = posterior left ventricular wall.

The term "scan" will be used frequently throughout this manual and denotes a change in angulation of the transducer from one cardiac structure to another while the paper records continuously. Figure 12*A* graphically illustrates the transducer's being directed toward mitral valve structures (position 1); then with slow, continuous motion, the transducer is tilted toward position 4, the ultrasound beam being directed into aortic and left atrial structures. If the paper was recording throughout the scan, a hard copy will have been made of all the intracardiac structures transected and their variability of motion. Of course a scan may be recorded from any direction as long as the identity of the structures being recorded is known.

Normal Mitral Valve

The mitral valve may be located by palpating the right ventricular outflow tract along the left sternal border. The transducer should then be placed perpendicularly on this pulsation and tilted slightly medially and cephalad. Probably only the anterior mitral leaflet will be visualized on the oscilloscope as a pattern of motion resembling an "M." The posterior mitral leaflet may then be found by the slightest tilt of the transducer inferiorly and laterally. Too much angulation will not position the sound beam over the posterior leaflet properly, and the expected motion—which is the opposite of that of the anterior leaflet—will not be seen.

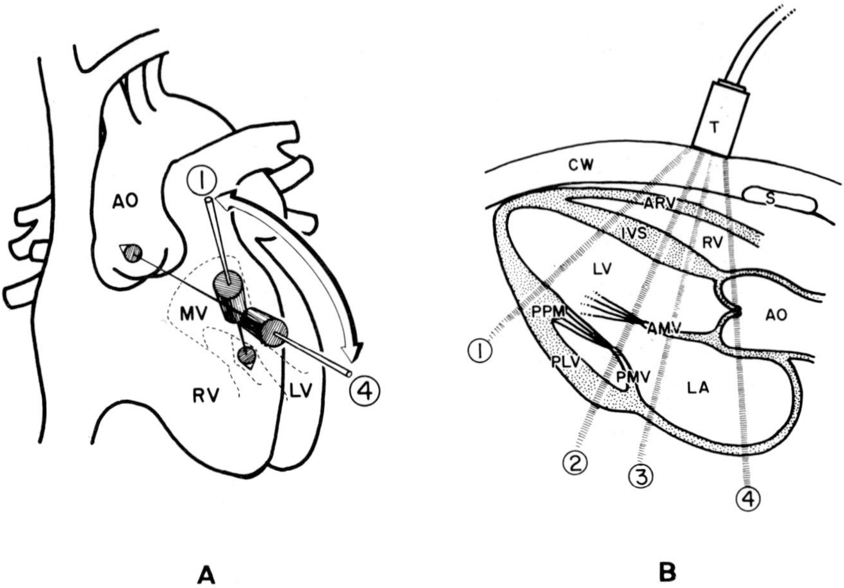

Figure 12. *A*, Angulation of transducer from mitral position to aortic position; *B*, structures transected as transducer is angled from mitral valve area to aorta. AO=aorta, MV=mitral valve, RV=right ventricle, LV=left ventricle, CW=chest wall, T=transducer, ARV=anterior right ventricular wall, PPM=posterior papillary muscle, PLV=posterior left ventricular wall, AMV=anterior mitral valve, PMV=posterior mitral valve, LA=left atrium, S=sternum and IVS=interventricular septum. (From Feigenbaum, H.: Clinical applications of echocardiography. Prog. Cardiovasc. Dis., *14*:531, 1972. By permission of Grune and Stratton, Inc.)

Both anterior and posterior mitral leaflets should be well defined. The more perpendicular the ultrasound beam is to the leaflets, the stronger and more solid will be the pattern of motion returned from the valve. The pattern of motion should appear unbroken and as complete as possible from the onset (D) to the end of diastole when the mitral valve closes (C in Figure 13).

Multiple echoes may be seen originating from the mitral leaflets. Since the mitral valve is not a perfectly flat reflecting interface and the sound beam has some lateral width, echoes from many parts of the valve are returned simultaneously. These echoes should not be mistaken for thickening of the valve structure.

One should be able to see the mitral leaflets separate from each other with the onset of diastole, stay open as long as passive ventricular filling occurs and close after atrial contraction (A in Figure 13). The transducer should be tilted up or down the valve while continuously recording to obtain the maximum cusps' separation. Maximum cusps' separation is identified by E–E′ (Figure 13). At this time rapid ventricular filling begins. The greatest volume of blood passes from the

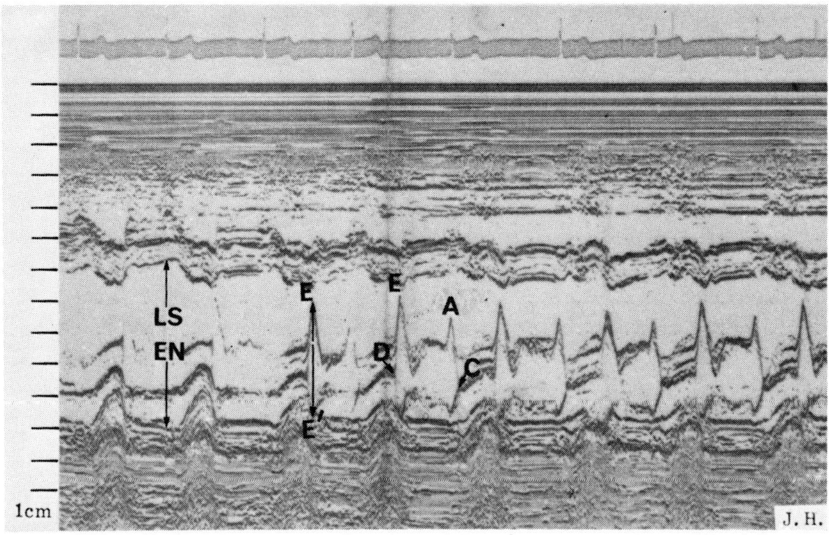

Figure 13. Normal mitral valve, scanned from chordal attachments toward atrioventricular junction. LS = left side of septum, EN = endocardial surface of posterior left ventricular wall, E = maximum opening point of anterior mitral leaflet, E′ = maximum opening point of posterior mitral leaflet, D = initial point of opening of mitral valve, C = closure of the mitral valve and A = peak of atrial contraction prior to closure of mitral valve.

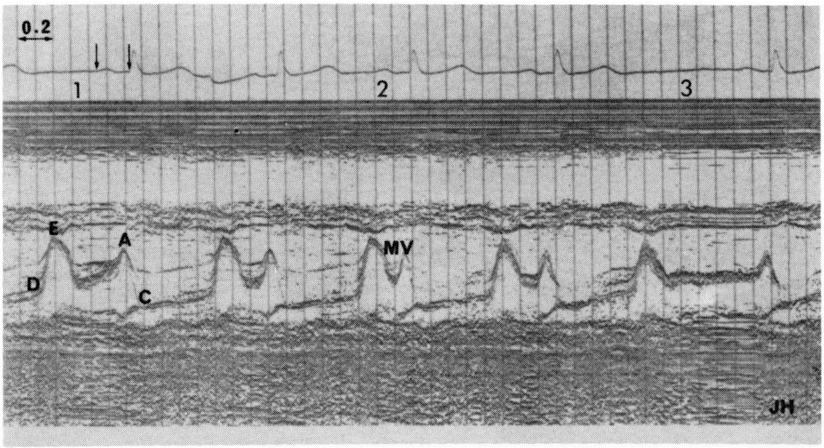

Figure 14. Normal mitral valve exhibiting effects of sinus arrhythmia. D = initial opening of mitral valve during rapid ventricular filling, E = maximum opening amplitude of anterior mitral leaflet, A = peak of atrial contraction, C = closure of mitral valve and MV = mitral valve. Arrows denote P–R interval on electrocardiogram.

left atrium through the leaflets into the left ventricle. The separation of these leaflets may be directly related to the quantity and velocity of blood passing through them.

The cusps' separation of the normal mitral valve may vary from 2.6 to 3.7 cm, the amount of separation noted in a study of 130 subjects without evidence of disease. Should either the cardiac output or the velocity of flow be reduced, the leaflets may be expected to separate less, usually from 1.9 to 2.5 cm. Should the cardiac output through the mitral valve be increased, the leaflets may separate 3.9 to 5.0 cm. Patients with significant mitral insufficiency without obstruction and high output states have cusp separation above the normal limits.

The pattern of the mitral valve motion may vary from one diastolic cycle to the next, depending on the length of the diastolic period. Figure 14 shows five mitral complexes in a normal individual with sinus arrhythmia. The diastolic period of complexes 1, 2 and 3 are all different, thus changing the configuration of the pattern of motion of the valve. However, this is not an indication of mitral valve dysfunction but only reflects the variability of time elapsed during diastole and the valve's response to passive blood flow.

Mitral Stenosis

Obstruction of the mitral valve, as resulting from mitral stenosis, causes the two cusps of the valve to move in the same direction, *i.e.*, toward the transducer with the onset of diastole (Figure 15). Frequently the posterior mitral valve appears to be stationary, or it will only move a slight amount. The anterior mitral valve exhibits the most excursion and is evaluated for amplitude of motion, thickness and closing velocity.

The amplitude of opening of the anterior mitral cusp varies according to where the ultrasound beam transects the structure. If the beam passes through the valve at the level of the chordal attachments, the valve appears to have reduced opening amplitude, but as the angle of the transducer is changed, tilting toward the left atrium while continuously recording, the amplitude of the valve steadily increases. At the point where the posterior leaflet almost drops out of the tracing, measurements of the valve should be taken.

Figure 16 is a slightly different view of the same valve seen in Figure 15. The closing velocity of the valve is calculated to be 15 mm/sec, which places it in the range of moderate mitral stenosis. The opening amplitude of the leaflet measures 28 mm, indicating a pliable valve. This has not been proven to be an indication of the size of the orifice. The anterior and posterior leaflets appear to be generally but not densely thickened, as would be apparent with heavy fibrosis or calcification.

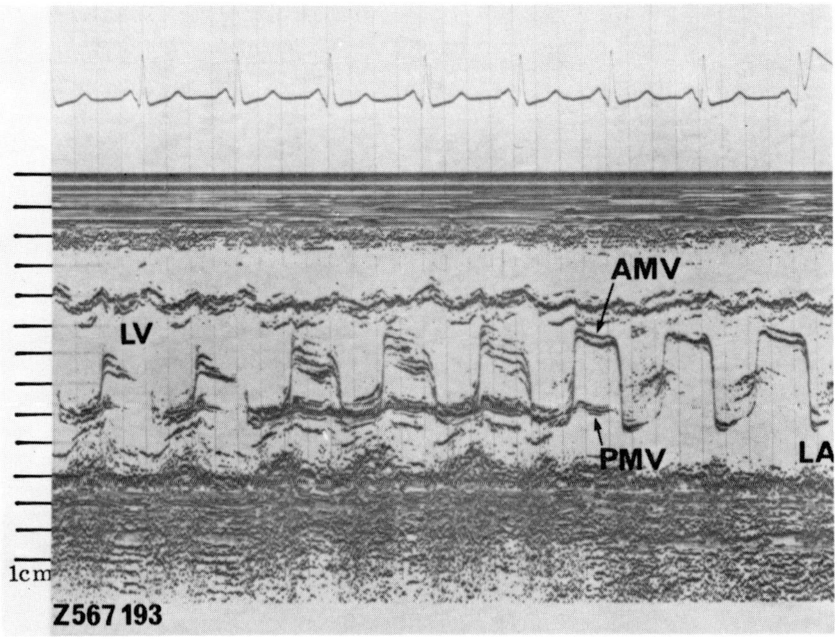

Figure 15. Valve configuration seen with mitral stenosis. LV = left ventricle, AMV = anterior mitral valve, PMV = posterior mitral valve and LA = left atrium.

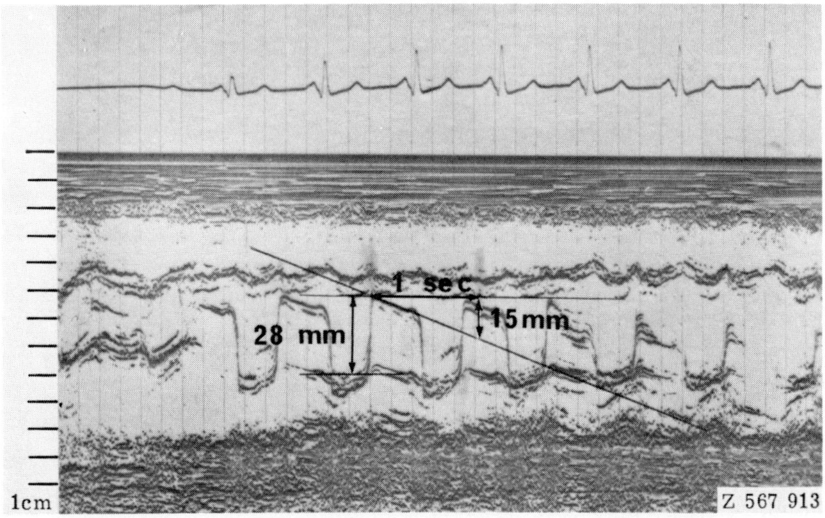

Figure 16. Parameters used to evaluate amount of mitral valve obstruction. Catheterization data show this valve to have an orifice of 1.2 cm^2, cardiac index of 3.7 L/min/M^2 and no evidence of mitral insufficiency. The resting mitral valve gradient was 40 mm Hg. A successful mitral commissurotomy was performed.

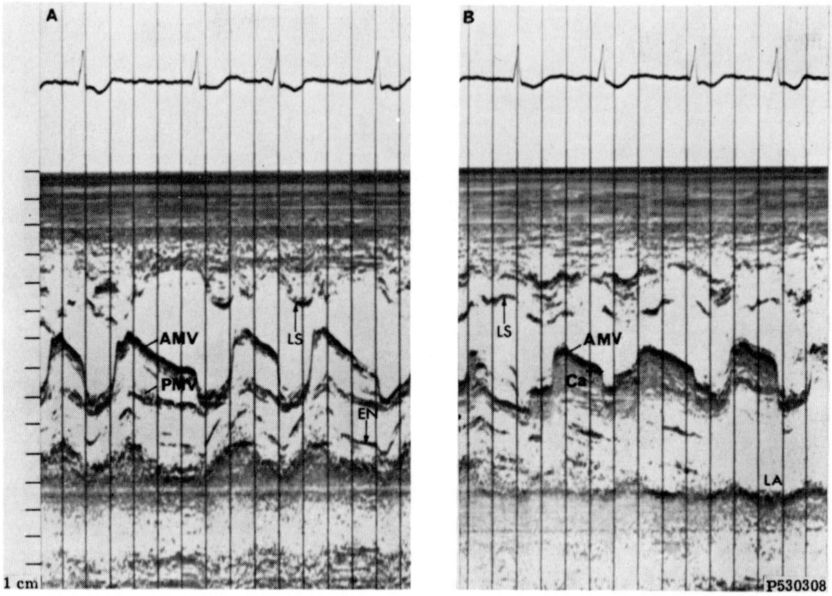

Figure 17. *A*, Mitral stenosis without evidence of calcification; *B*, same valve, recorded from a more superior plane, *i.e.*, transducer was pointed toward atrium. Dense echoes under anterior mitral leaflet during diastole represent areas of calcification. Gain settings between tracings *A* and *B* were not altered. AMV = anterior mitral valve, PMV = posterior mitral valve, LS = left septum, EN = endocardial surface of posterior left ventricular wall, Ca^{++} = calcium and LA = left atrium.

Calcified Mitral Valve with Stenosis

Great care should be taken when scanning the mitral leaflet from the chordal attachments to the annular attachment. Often areas of calcification or dense fibrosis may not be seen in one portion of the leaflet (Figure 17*A*) but by redirecting the sound beam, the valve becomes heavily echo-producing (Figure 17*B*). It is reported that the ultrasound is more sensitive to calcification and dense fibrosis than is fluoroscopy.

One should experiment with different gain settings during an examination of the leaflets. If excessive echoes are present, even at very low gain settings, evidence for calcification or dense fibrosis should be noted.

Figure 18 shows a routine scan from left ventricle to left atrium. The mitral valve is seen to be heavily echo-producing in the area of the anterior and posterior mitral leaflets; in fact the leaflets become almost indistinguishable from each other owing to the amount of calcium present. The left atrial dimension is markedly dilated.

Catheterization data disclosed severe mitral stenosis and moderate

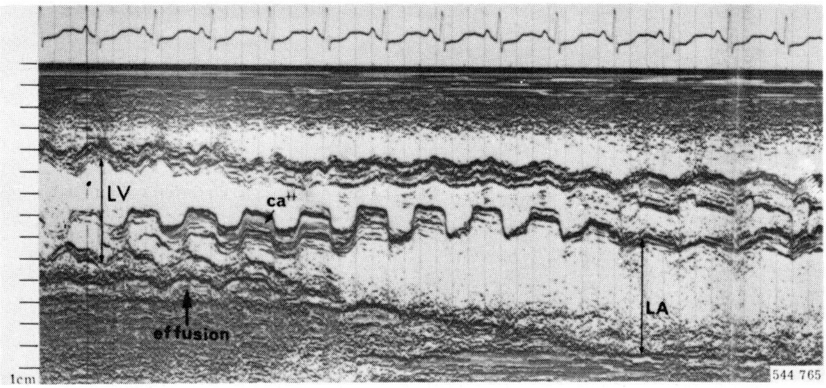

Figure 18. Routine M-mode scan from left ventricle to left atrium. Mitral valve is heavily calcified and opens poorly. LA = left atrium and Ca^{++} = calcium and LV = left ventricle.

mitral insufficiency. Pulmonary pressures were elevated at rest and rose to systemic levels during exercise. The patient was referred for surgical replacement of the mitral valve. Recovery from the operative procedure was uneventful and essentially uncomplicated except for persistent atrial fibrillation.

Mitral Stenosis Following Commissurotomy

Figure 19*A* is from a patient with moderately severe, noncalcific mitral stenosis. The posterior mitral leaflet moves in the same direction as the anterior mitral leaflet with the onset of diastole. Following mitral commissurotomy, the closing velocity of the mitral valve was greatly increased (Figure 19*B*). The posterior mitral leaflet moves almost normally: an excellent surgical result.

Occasionally the posterior leaflet of the mitral valve will be seen to move in a normal pattern following surgical treatment. This is not to assume that mitral stenosis is no longer present. Thickening of the anterior mitral valve is still present and the closing velocity of the leaflet is still reduced, although it may be improved over the preoperative condition. Figure 20 demonstrates a thickened anterior mitral leaflet with reduced velocity of closure and a normally moving posterior leaflet. Similar tracings from other patients are reported in the literature.

False Mitral Stenosis

Figure 21 was recorded as soon as the transducer was placed on the patient's chest, along the left sternal border. At first glance the patient seemed to have mitral stenosis and a normally moving tricuspid valve. However, further examination revealed no posterior mitral cusp, and the left ventricle was exceedingly difficult to locate.

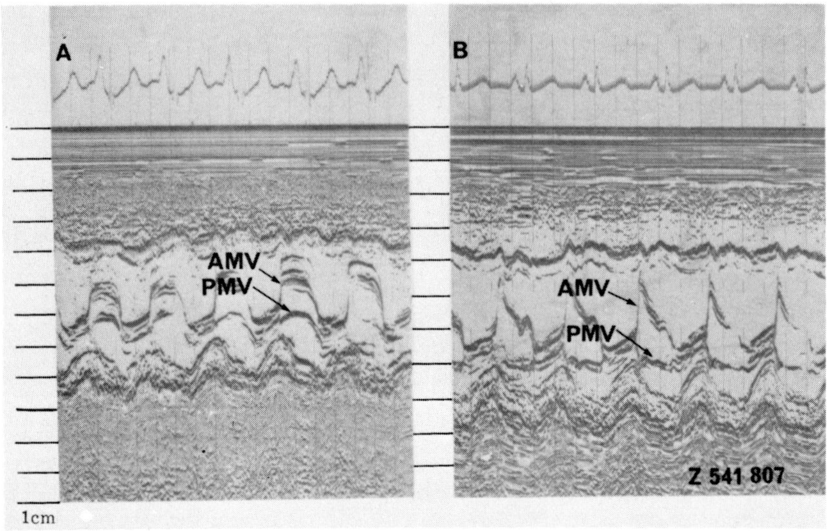

Figure 19. *A,* Mitral stenosis before surgical intervention. Closing velocity of mitral valve is greatly reduced; *B,* same mitral valve postoperatively prior to patient's discharge from hospital. Closing velocity of mitral valve is greatly improved and posterior leaflet moves more normally. AMV = anterior mitral valve and PMV = posterior mitral valve.

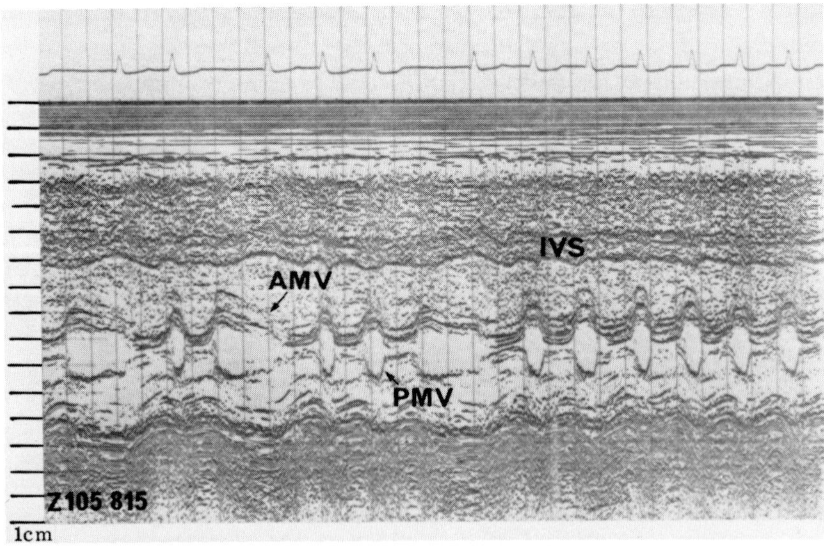

Figure 20. Postoperative tracing of mitral valve showing normal motion of posterior leaflet and typical stenotic pattern on anterior leaflet. Preoperative tracings were not done. Mitral commissurotomy was performed in 1962. AMV = anterior mitral valve, PMV = posterior mitral valve and IVS = interventricular septum.

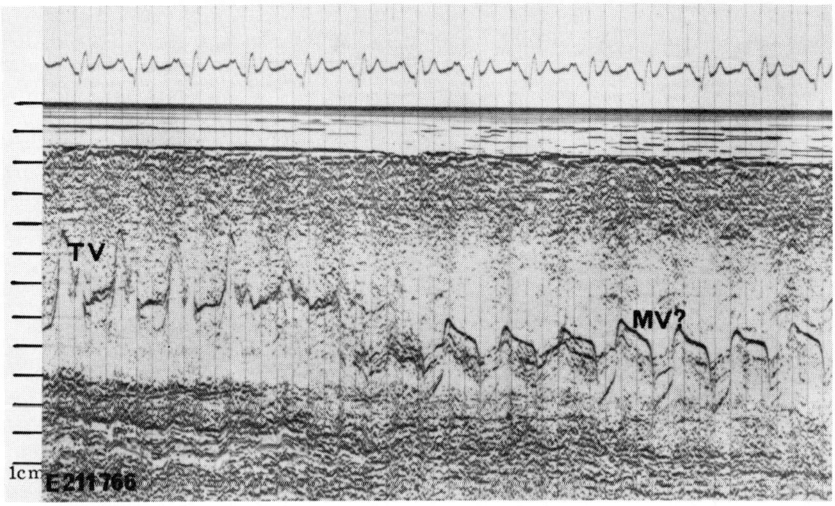

Figure 21. Initial recording made on patient on whom preliminary diagnosis of transposition, dextroversion and pulmonary stenosis was made. TV = tricuspid valve and MV = mitral valve.

There was a short interlude while the examiner consulted the chart to determine why mitral stenosis had not been noted and to obtain a clue as to the location of the left ventricle. Dextroversion being noted, the transducer was then positioned along the left sternal border and directed *superiorly and laterally* toward the left shoulder. The mitral valve was recorded from this position and was noted to move normally (Figure 22). What was previously thought to be the mitral valve was actually a large pulmonary valve; recorded directly in line and superior to this valve was a smaller arterial valve, the aortic valve. Recording these two arterial valves simultaneously in this 19-year-old patient indicated transposition of the great vessels (Figure 22). The motion of the pulmonary valve was consistent with pulmonary hypertension but not with pulmonary stenosis (see pp. 77–79).

The main lesson to be learned from this patient is that patterns of motion may represent one disease and actually be something entirely different. Before completing any examination, the examiner should be sure that all the anatomical structures have been correctly identified.

Bacterial Endocarditis Vegetations

The question is, how do we distinguish between calcific thickening and vegetations on the mitral valve? Calcium or dense fibrosis is usually associated with mitral stenosis. Vegetations from subacute bacterial

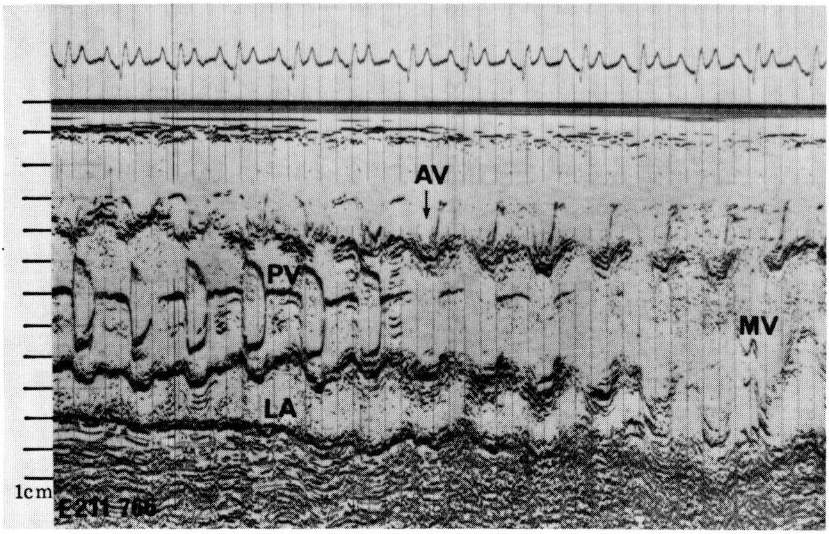

Figure 22. Final tracing on 19-year-old white male with echocardiographic evidence of transposition of great vessels. PV = pulmonary valve, AV = aortic valve, LA = left atrium and MV = mitral valve.

endocarditis (SBE) or markedly roughened and irregular leaflet surfaces resulting from rheumatic heart disease or myxomatous degeneration appear as thickened areas on a very mobile valve.

Unless the thickening is obvious, however, it would be better to underread this event. One may monitor the patient with serial echograms to see if the echoes increase. We have patients in whom the areas of possible vegetative process have not shown progression of leaflet thickening on the echogram. However, the leaflets were being damaged to the point of becoming perforated or flail, these states being identified at time of surgical treatment.

Figure 23 illustrates our major problem of identifying all the abnormalities that may be present. These leaflets appear thickened, and vegetations of the anterior leaflet were suspected. At no time did we see echocardiographic evidence of a flail posterior mitral leaflet. The left atrium is dilated as is the left ventricle.

Eventually this patient so deteriorated that surgical intervention was required. The anterior leaflet was not flail. The pathology report noted that the edges of the mitral leaflets were markedly thickened and irregular. The surface was rough, and near the edge friable vegetation was noted. No pericardial effusion was noted, but there was a large left pleural effusion. The surgery report described the mitral valve as follows: "The posterior mural leaflet was completely flail. One part of the posterior leaflet, near its center, had a slender portion which flopped back and forth freely and had vegetations on it and looked

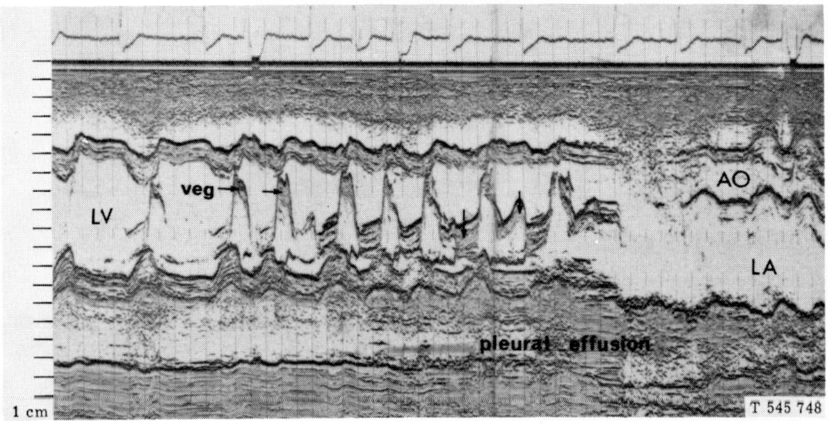

Figure 23. Scan from left ventricle through mitral valve into left atrium and aorta. As scan moves from low mitral valve to its annular attachment, many different planes of anterior cusp are recorded. Thickening thus may be seen on valve during systole and diastole, no two complexes looking exactly alike. Veg = vegetations, LV = left ventricle, AO = aorta and LA = left atrium.

pretty clearly as if it had resulted from perforations along either side. There was an additional large perforation nearby in this leaflet. There was, furthermore, one easily identified perforation in the septal leaflet. The cords were all intact and seemed to be fibrotic."

Figure 24 is from a patient who was referred for an echocardiographic consultation to evaluate mitral insufficiency and to determine vegetations on the mitral valve. The routine study of the mitral valve did not disclose any unusual thickening of the anterior or posterior mitral leaflets. The only abnormality noted was prolapsing of the posterior mitral leaflet (arrow).

However, as the transducer was angled toward the left atrium (Fig. 25), the anterior mitral leaflet was seen to have thickened material hanging from the leaflet, its appearance changing as the angle of the transducer was changed. This was determined to be a mass of material, possibly vegetative. The patient was subsequently taken to cardiac catheterization. Data from that study confirmed severe mitral insufficiency, and the patient was referred for mitral valve replacement.

Surgical description of this diseased mitral valve was noted in the patient's hospital chart as follows: "It was seen that the minor or posterior leaflet was intact and normal. All chordae were present and supporting the valve leaflet. The major leaflet had broken chordae on the caudal aspect and at approximately the junction of the cephalad ¾ of the valve and the caudal ¼. Approximately 3–4 mm from the edge of the leaflet, there was a vegetation that appeared to be 5 mm long, 4 mm wide, and 3 mm thick; the lack of support for the valve was in this area where chordae had been fractured."

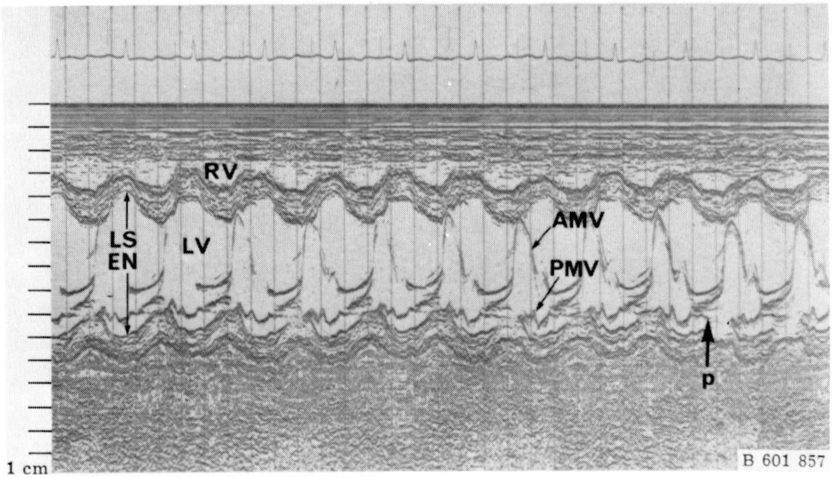

Figure 24. Usual view of mitral valve when transducer is directed into left ventricle. Only prolapsing of posterior mitral leaflet is noted. RV = right ventricle, LV = left ventricle, LS = left septum, EN = endocardium, AMV = anterior mitral valve, PMV = posterior mitral valve and p = prolapse.

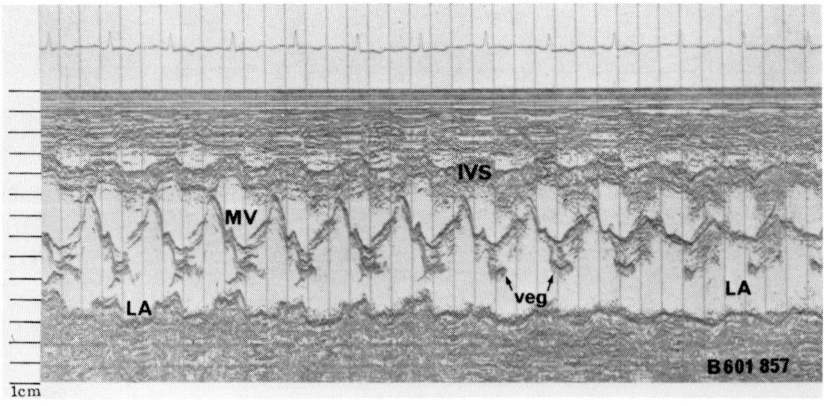

Figure 25. Mitral valve with vegetations. Transducer has been directed toward left atrium. Posterior mitral leaflet is not well visualized. LA=left atrium, veg=vegetations, MV=mitral valve, IVS=interventricular septum.

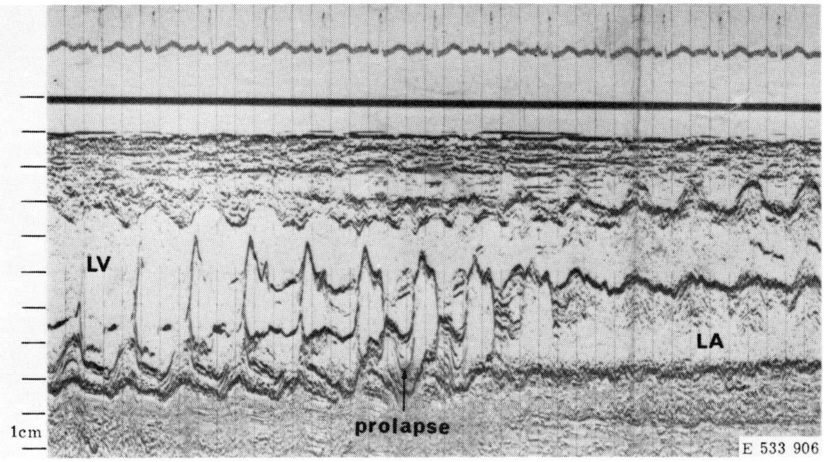

Figure 26. Prolapsing mitral valve, visualized at atrioventricular junction. LV = left ventricle and LA = left atrium.

Prolapsed Mitral Valve

Many prolapsed mitral leaflets, especially those of a minor degree, are missed because the full posterior leaflet excursion was never recorded.

There are two approaches to recording prolapses. The more common one utilizes a full scan of the mitral valve. The patient is positioned somewhat left laterally, and his head and torso are elevated to approximately 30°. Other examiners prefer to have the patient sitting. The transducer is angled from the free edges of the mitral leaflets to the annular attachment. As the transducer is angled from the left ventricle toward the left atrium, the prolapse is most often seen at the junction between the two chambers (Figure 26).

The main disadvantage of this approach is that the late systolic motion of the posterior leaflet is obscured by the anteriorly moving posterior left ventricular wall. It is essential to angle the transducer high enough to clear the left ventricular wall and to be positioned in a plane with the lower left atrial wall.

The second and preferred approach is to find the mitral valve from one higher intercostal space. This may necessitate angling the transducer slightly inferiorly and medially, but now both leaflets may be seen clearly outlined against the lower left atrial wall which lies posterior to the leaflets (Figure 27).

Sometimes one may see a variation in the opening amplitude of the prolapsing mitral valve with respiration. Complex 1 in Figure 27 shows the mitral valve opening with full amplitude; complex 2 shows the effect of reduced blood flow through the valve when the patient exhaled more vigorously than usual, thus creating a mini-Valsalva maneuver.

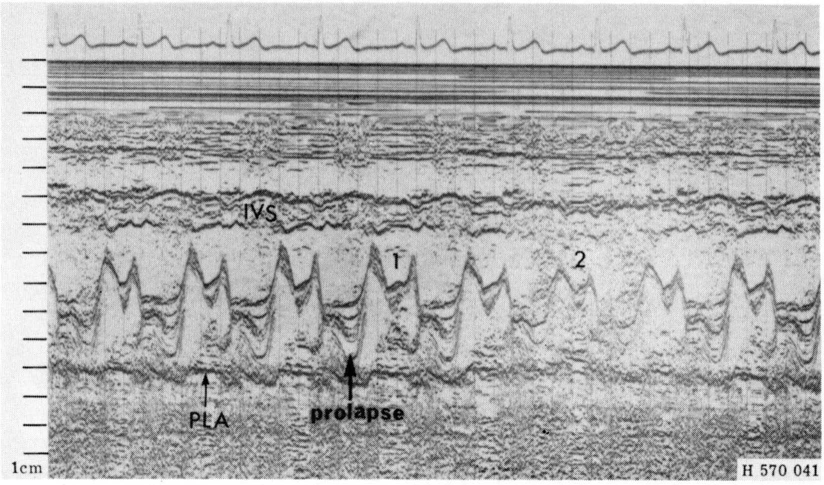

Figure 27. Prolapsed mitral valve recorded from one intercostal space higher than that from which remainder of study was recorded. IVS = interventricular septum, PLA = posterior left atrial wall, 1 = mitral complex during quiet inspiration and 2 = mitral complex during vigorous expiration.

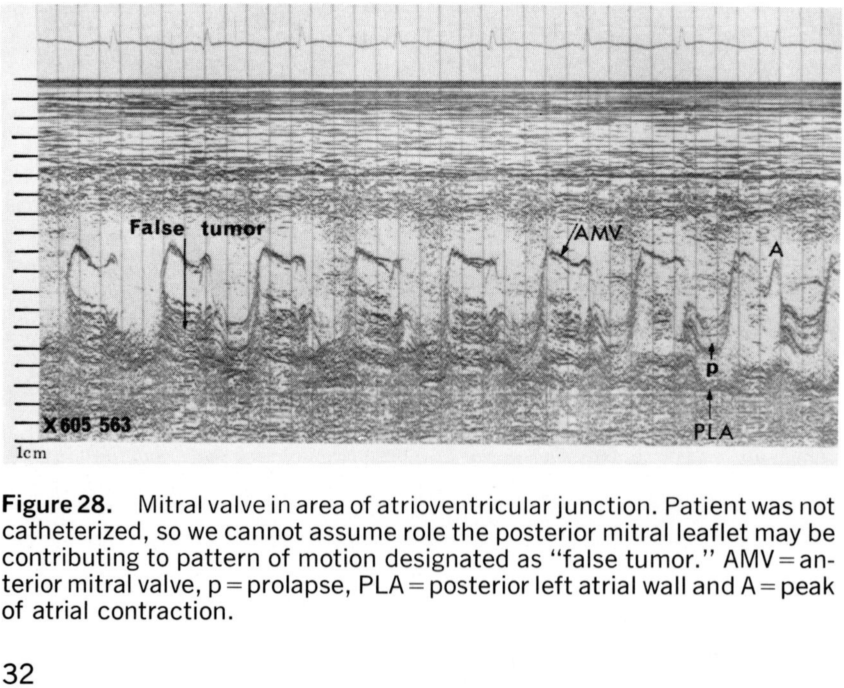

Figure 28. Mitral valve in area of atrioventricular junction. Patient was not catheterized, so we cannot assume role the posterior mitral leaflet may be contributing to pattern of motion designated as "false tumor." AMV = anterior mitral valve, p = prolapse, PLA = posterior left atrial wall and A = peak of atrial contraction.

Mitral Prolapse Mimicking Stenosis and Left Atrial Tumor

Scanning the mitral valve from the chordal attachments toward the annulus is a necessary technique to rule out a variety of pattern motions simulating one or more types of mitral disease.

Figure 28 shows the mitral valve in the area of the atrioventricular junction just before the ultrasound beam passes into the left atrium. The closing velocity of the mitral valve is reduced but shows a definite atrial contraction. The posterior leaflet seems to be obscured by a mass of echoes labeled "false tumor." By scanning higher into the left atrium, it is observed that the anterior leaflet exhibits classic prolapsing of the mitral valve.

Figure 29 was recorded from patient described in Figure 28. The transducer was angled from the left atrium and aorta, inferiorly toward the mitral valve. The left atrium is now seen to be empty of any organized echoes, and none is seen under the anterior mitral leaflet. The proper echocardiographic interpretation on this patient should read as severe prolapsing of the mitral valve. The complete examination revealed no evidence for left atrial myxoma or mitral stenosis. This patient is described as having Marfan's syndrome.

Left Atrial Myxoma (Tumor)

Left atrial myxomas can mimic mitral stenosis. The opening amplitude of the mitral valve is normal; the closing velocity of the valve is reduced; and the left atrium is dilated. However, there appears to be a space-occupying mass, which does not resemble calcium or dense fibrosis, situated under the anterior leaflet (Figure 30). It is the

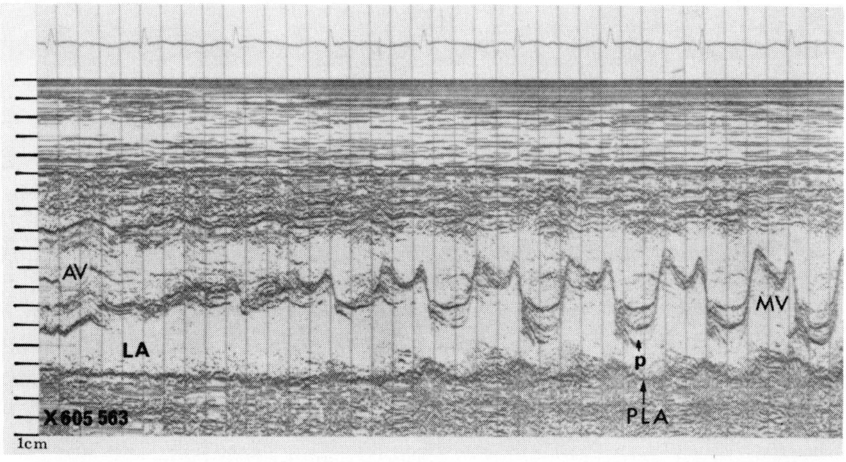

Figure 29. Scan from aorta to mitral valve. There is no evidence of space-occupying mass in left atrium or under anterior mitral leaflet. AV = aortic valve, LA = left atrium, p = prolapse, PLA = posterior left atrial wall and MV = mitral valve.

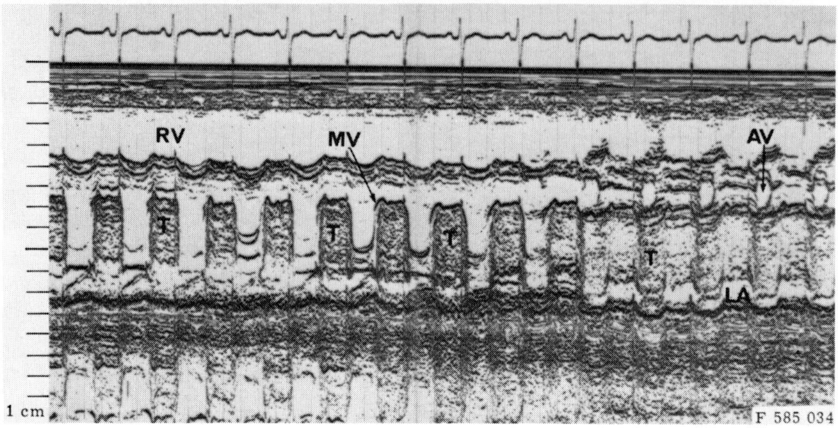

Figure 30. Left atrial myxoma. RV = right ventricle, T = tumor, MV = mitral valve, AV = aortic valve and LA = left atrium.

obligation of the examiner to determine if this mass is attributable to too much gain or if it is real tissue.

In Figure 30 the gain has been reduced to levels that are adequate to visualize the septum and posterior wall without difficulty. The tumor, which is shown as an organized mass of echoes under the mitral leaflet, is not obliterated by low gain settings. One should notice the slight delay between the time the mitral valve opens and the time the tumor enters the mitral orifice. By scanning toward the left atrium, one can record the tumor prolapsing back into that chamber during systole. This tumor was an exceptionally large one, nearly filling the left atrial chamber.

Following removal of the tumor, the anterior mitral valve is seen to move normally without evidence of obstruction or thickening of the leaflets (Figure 31). The posterior leaflet, which was not seen preoperatively, is now visible and moves normally. Preoperatively the posterior leaflet had been obscured by the tumor entering the mitral orifice.

In most cases these tumors are benign and do not recur. If recurrence takes place, the pattern for tumors interfering with normal valve motion would again reappear, as was seen once at the Indiana University Laboratory. The patient had a rhabdomyosarcoma. Serial examination of the mitral valve for 3 months postoperatively again showed the typical echocardiographic pattern for tumor.

Normal Left Ventricular End-diastolic Pressure (LVEDp)

When a patient is being evaluated for left ventricular dysfunction, one becomes concerned with the measurement of left ventricular end-diastolic pressure. Reports in the literature indicate that echocar-

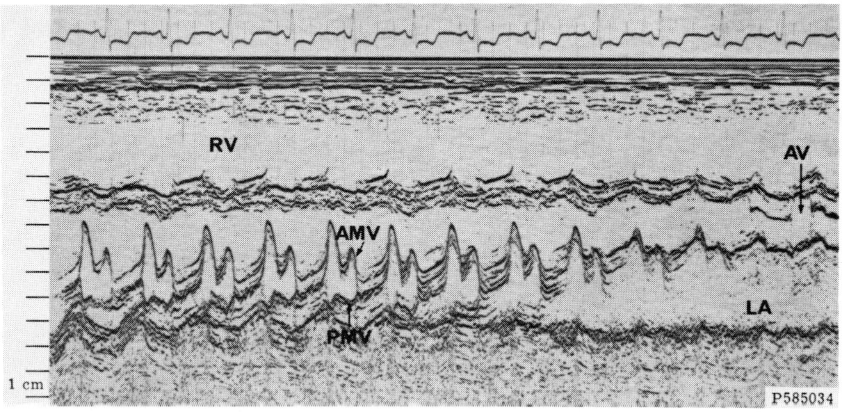

Figure 31. Postoperative scan after removal of left atrial myxoma. RV = right ventricle, AMV = anterior mitral leaflet, PMV = posterior mitral valve, AV = aortic valve and LA = left atrium.

diography can detect the difference between normal and elevated left ventricular end-diastolic pressure based on the time it takes the mitral valve to close. It is therefore important for the examiner to obtain as nearly perfect a mitral valve tracing as possible, especially between atrial contraction to closure. The proper measurements cannot be made unless the two cusps of the mitral valve are seen to *meet* at what has been designated as the "C" point (Figure 32). As Dr. Feigenbaum, in his book *Echocardiography,* states ". . . the measurement taken is the P–R minus A–C interval. Normally, the P–R interval is 0.06 sec. greater than the A–C interval. A P–R minus A–C interval of 0.06 sec. or less indicates that the left ventricular end-diastolic pressure is at least 20 mm Hg and the atrial component of the left ventricular pressure is at least 8 mm Hg."

For ease of measuring, recording paper speed may be set at 50 to 100 mm/sec, and the time-line intervals set at 0.1 or 0.04 sec. Paper speeds of 25 mm/sec and time-line intervals of 0.2 sec are too slow to make accurate measurements.

Elevated Left Ventricular End-diastolic Pressure

The atrial contraction in Figure 33 can be seen more easily on the posterior leaflet of the mitral valve. This is especially true if the cardiac output is markedly reduced, as it is here. The cusps are separating 2.7 cm, which is at the lower normal limits.

The atrial contraction seen on the mitral valve should be timed with the electrocardiogram to identify correctly the proper "A" wave; P–R minus A–C in Figure 33 is equal to 0.06 sec. This is a borderline measurement and by common practice is considered to be abnormal and therefore indicative of elevated left ventricular end-diastolic pressure as confirmed at catheterization.

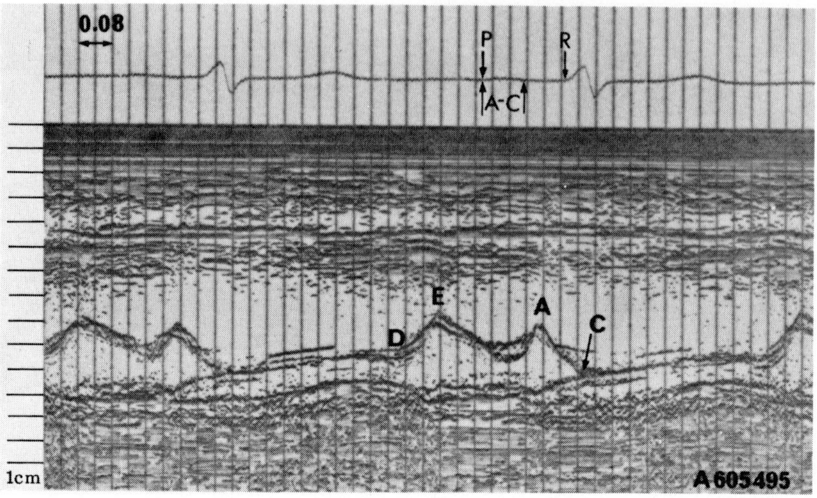

Figure 32. Mitral valve with normal closure. Paper recording speed was 100 mm/sec and time-line intervals were set at 0.04 sec. D = initial opening of mitral valve, E = maximum opening of mitral valve, A = peak of atrial contraction, C = closure of anterior and posterior mitral cusps.

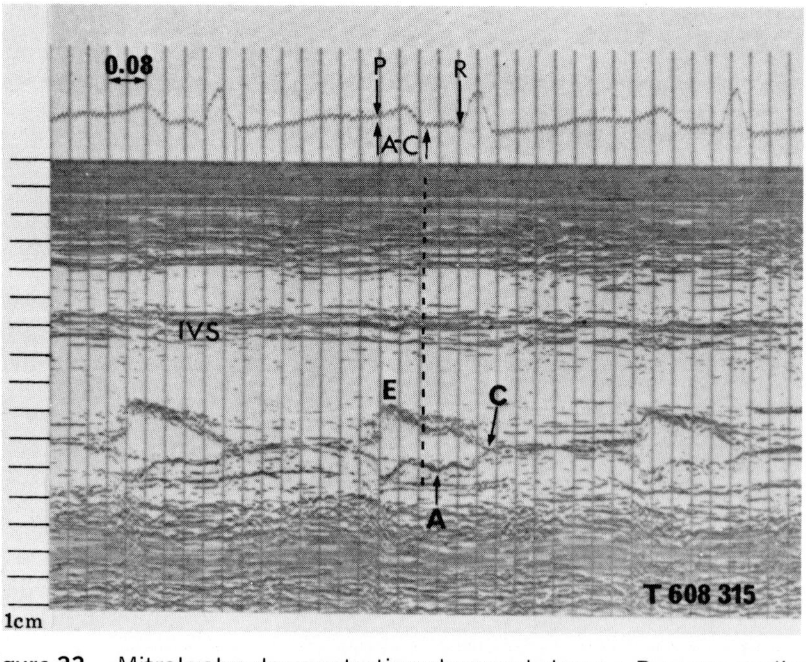

Figure 33. Mitral valve demonstrating abnormal closure. Paper recording speed was 100 mm/sec with time-line intervals of 0.04 sec. IVS = interventricular septum, E = maximum opening of mitral valve, A = peak of atrial contraction and C = closure of both cusps of mitral valve.

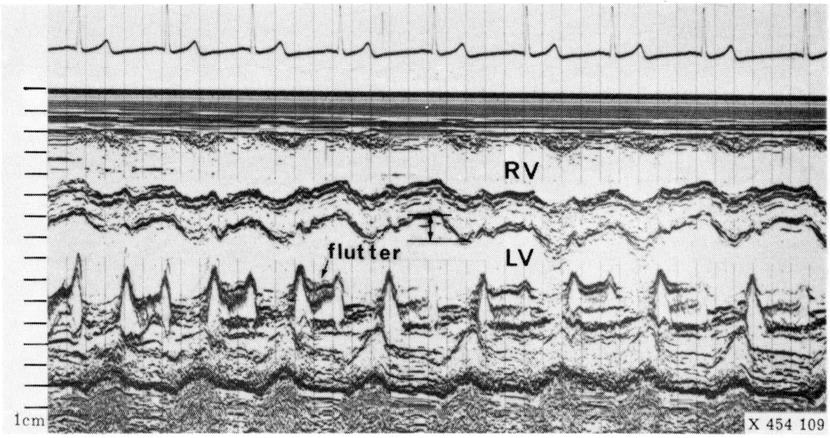

Figure 34. Fluttering of mitral valve in presence of significant aortic insufficiency. Amount of fluttering is not indicative of extent of insufficiency. RV = right ventricle and LV = left ventricle.

Aortic Insufficiency and Mitral Valve Motion

Extremely fine oscillations of the mitral valve as seen in Figure 34 are attributable to the jet of aortic insufficiency striking the mitral valve, causing the leaflet to vibrate. The aortic regurgitant jet may also be mixing with the normal inflow of blood from the left atrium into the left ventricle. This mixing of blood from two different directions causes an area of turbulence in which the leaflets vibrate or "flutter."

Diastolic closing velocities and cusps' separation of the mitral valve should not be measured when the physiological motion is significantly altered by the effects of aortic insufficiency. The figures obtained will not be accurate.

Aortic insufficiency may cause reduced closing velocity of the anterior mitral leaflet; one may then misinterpret this pattern of motion as mitral stenosis (Figure 35). Examination of the tracing reveals the leaflets to be thin and pliable. The posterior mitral leaflet moves away from the transducer with the onset of diastole and responds well to atrial contraction. The only abnormality noted is the fine fluttering of the anterior mitral leaflet during diastole. Mitral stenosis is absent.

Acute Aortic Insufficiency

The patient whose mitral valve is illustrated in Figure 36 developed acute aortic insufficiency, a fatal condition if surgical intervention is not prompt. The initial closure of the mitral valve takes place well before diastole is over and the valve remains effectively closed through the latter part of diastole. Fluttering of the mitral leaflet is not common.

During surgical repair the aortic valve was seen to be bicuspid with a

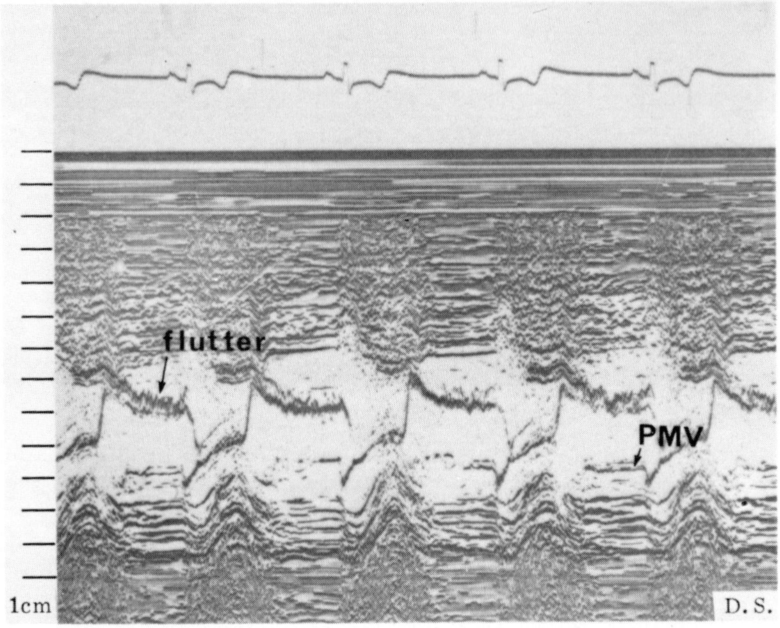

Figure 35. Mitral valve mimicking mitral stenosis. "Flutter" vibrations on anterior mitral leaflet are caused by regurgitant jet of aortic blood striking leaflet during diastole. Auscultation revealed an Austin-Flint murmur. Normal motion of posterior mitral leaflet and general "thinness" of leaflets rule out mitral stenosis. PMV = posterior mitral valve.

rent in one of the leaflets; the valve exhibited mucoid degeneration and no vegetations were present on any of the leaflets. On the echocardiogram the aortic leaflets opened well and were not thickened, and no abnormal motion during systole was noted.

At this laboratory all of the patients with acute onset of aortic insufficiency with premature closure of the mitral valve have had surgical replacement of the aortic valve. If the patient has evidence of subacute bacterial endocarditis, he is monitored serially. As new murmurs develop, fluttering of the mitral valve may develop as the aortic valve degenerates.

It should be emphasized that the mitral valve is in no way diseased. Its motion merely reflects the hemodynamic changes taking place elsewhere in the heart.

Idiopathic Hypertrophic Subaortic Stenosis (IHSS)

Classic, obstructive IHSS causes the mitral valve to bulge forward against a thickened septum during systole (Figure 37, arrow). The more closely the systolic bulge of the mitral valve approximates the left

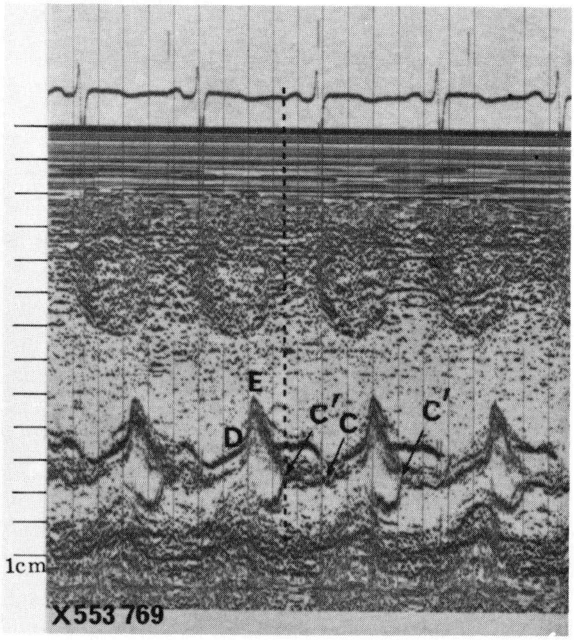

Figure 36. Mitral valve demonstrating acute aortic insufficiency. Valve is seen to close prematurely. E = maximum opening of mitral valve, C′ = premature closure of mitral valve and C = point at which mitral valve would normally close.

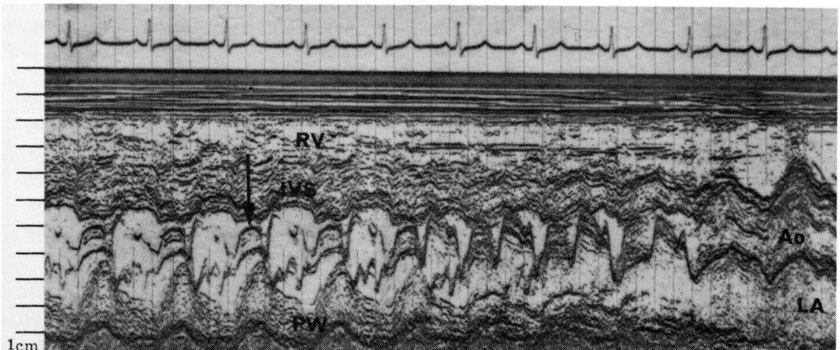

Figure 37. Mitral valve exhibiting systolic bulging against thickened interventricular septum. Mitral valve is not diseased but merely reflects abnormal motion into left ventricular outflow tract, possibly caused by Venturi effect. RV = right ventricle, IVS = interventricular septum, PW = posterior wall of left ventricle, Ao = aorta and LA = left atrium.

Table 1.
Provocative maneuvers to accentuate latent systolic obstruction

Provocation method	*Side effects*
Amyl nitrite inhalation	Increased heartrate, dizziness, peripheral flushing, seizures, fainting and headache
Hyperventilation	Dizziness, fainting, increased heartrate, anxiety and tingling in fingers
Carotid massage to provoke premature ventricular contractions	Slowing of heartrate, fainting and cardiac arrest

septum, the more obstruction there is to blood flowing into the left ventricular outflow tract toward the aorta.

At the time one is deciding whether or not the mitral valve shows systolic bulging, both leaflets of the valve should be seen. If the mitral annulus is recorded with some anterior mitral but no posterior leaflet, the impression may be that the anterior leaflet bulges. This is an artifact and should not even be regarded as a "false IHSS." The transducer should be angled deeper into the ventricle and both leaflets of the mitral valve should be recorded simultaneously before a judgment is made concerning the valve motion during systole.

If systolic bulging is not apparent in the presence of a thickened septum (known as ASH or asymmetrical septal hypertrophy), then some means of provocation must be used in an attempt to accentuate latent systolic obstruction. The patient may be challenged while both mitral leaflets are being recorded (Table 1). If a technician is initiating these procedures, a physician should be available during all the maneuvers, since serious side effects may occur.

Figure 38*A* was recorded from a patient with severe IHSS. The left ventricular outflow tract was almost totally obstructed during most of systole (arrow). At cardiac catheterization left ventricular pressures were measured above and below the site of obstruction, producing a resting gradient of 58 mm Hg and an exercise gradient of 84 mm Hg. The patient was given propranolol without symptomatic improvement and was referred for surgical correction.

Several months postoperatively Figure 38*B* shows the systolic bulging of the mitral valve to be considerably reduced and the left ventricular outflow tract no longer obstructed. Both sides of the septum are not well defined, and septal thickness could not be measured.

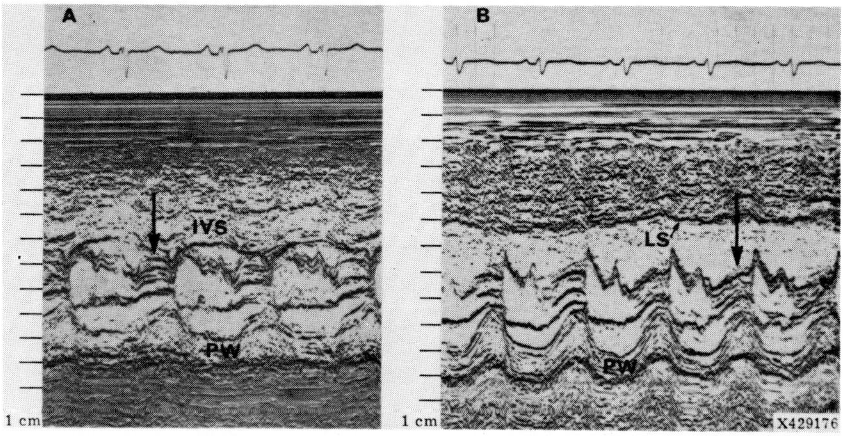

Figure 38. *A*, Preoperative, obstructive IHSS (arrow); *B*, echocardiogram obtained several months postmyomectomy. Systolic motion of mitral valve is still not entirely normal, but left ventricular outflow tract obstruction has been relieved (arrow). IVS = interventricular septum, PW = posterior left ventricular wall and LS = left septum.

Sufficient time should be allowed to elapse for healing to take place before judgments are made concerning the surgical result. Figure 39*A* was taken from a patient being considered for cardiac catheterization and operative intervention. The septum is thickened as is the posterior left ventricular wall. The systolic bulging of the mitral valve (arrow) completely obstructs the left ventricular outflow tract.

Before cardiac catheterization could be performed, the patient developed symptoms requiring emergency surgical intervention. An echocardiogram taken 2 days postoperatively revealed relief of the left ventricular outflow obstruction (Figure 39*B*). However, it was noted that the mitral cusps' separation was reduced, indicating diminished cardiac output, which would in turn cause reduction of the subaortic obstruction. Therefore the effects of the surgical maneuver could not be evaluated immediately postoperatively. The patient was subsequently discharged from hospital and has not returned for a follow-up echocardiogram.

Pseudo-IHSS

For unexplained reasons the mitral valve may exhibit systolic bulging mimicking IHSS in the absence of that disease. The septum may or may not be thickened, and the outflow tract of the left ventricle does not appear to be obstructed on the echogram. Provocation with amyl nitrite, hyperventilation, Valsalva maneuver and isoproterenol (Isuprel) did not produce gradients at cardiac catheterization (Figures 40–42).

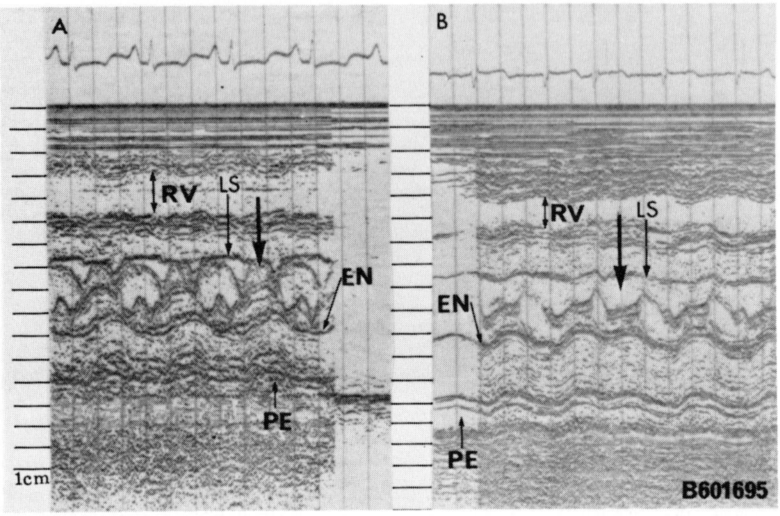

Figure 39. *A*, Preoperative echocardiogram of patient with severe, obstructive IHSS; *B*, postmyomectomy. Left ventricular outflow tract is less obstructed owing to reduced flow through mitral valve. RV = right ventricle, EN = endocardial surface of posterior left ventricular wall, LS = left septum and PE = pericardial effusion.

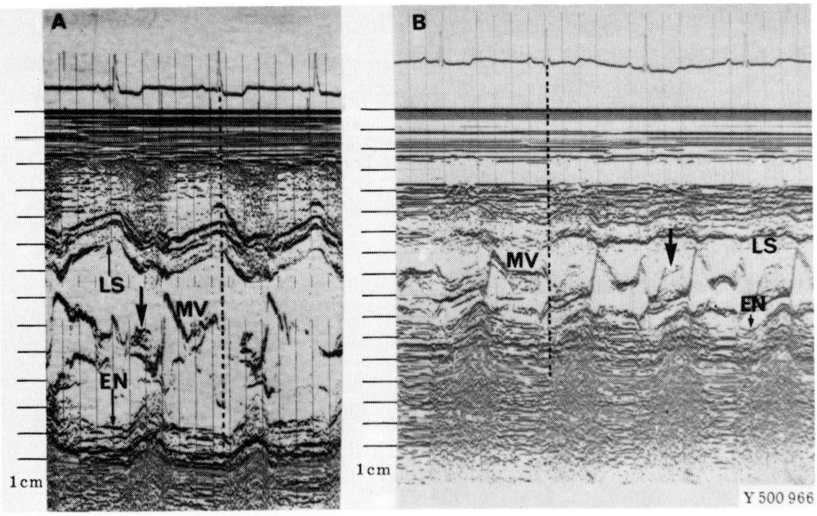

Figure 40. Patient, age 37, with moderately severe aortic insufficiency. *A*, Preoperative tracing showing flutter of mitral valve and pseudo-IHSS systolic bulging (large, unmarked arrow); *B*, postoperative tracing following aortic valve replacement. Pseudo-IHSS pattern is persistent. Abnormal septal motion following open-heart surgical procedure is common observance and has been reported in literature. LS = left septum, EN = endocardial surface of posterior left ventricular wall and MV = mitral valve.

Pseudo-IHSS–type motion has been observed in patients with aortic insufficiency (Figure 40), combined aortic stenosis, aortic insufficiency (Figure 41) and atrial septal defect (Figure 42).

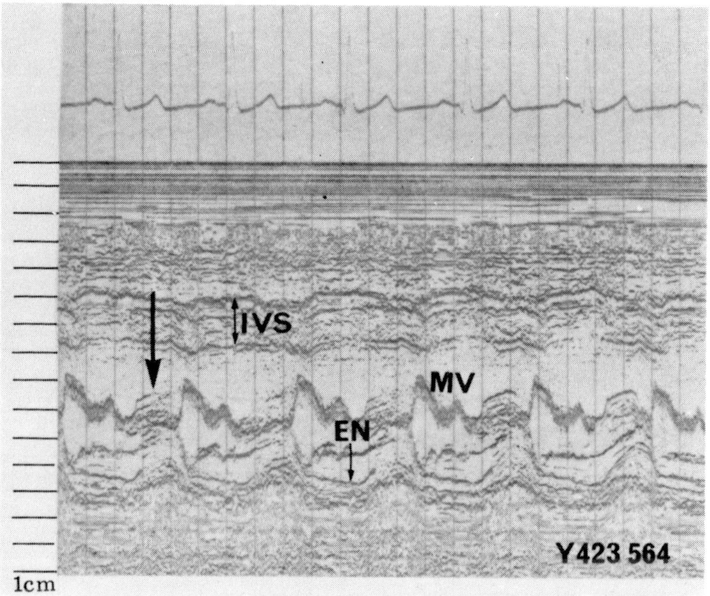

Figure 41. Patient with moderate aortic insufficiency and mild aortic stenosis exhibiting pseudo-IHSS systolic bulging of mitral valve. Fluttering mitral leaflet indicates aortic insufficiency. IVS = interventricular septum, EN = endocardial surface of posterior left ventricular wall and MV = mitral valve.

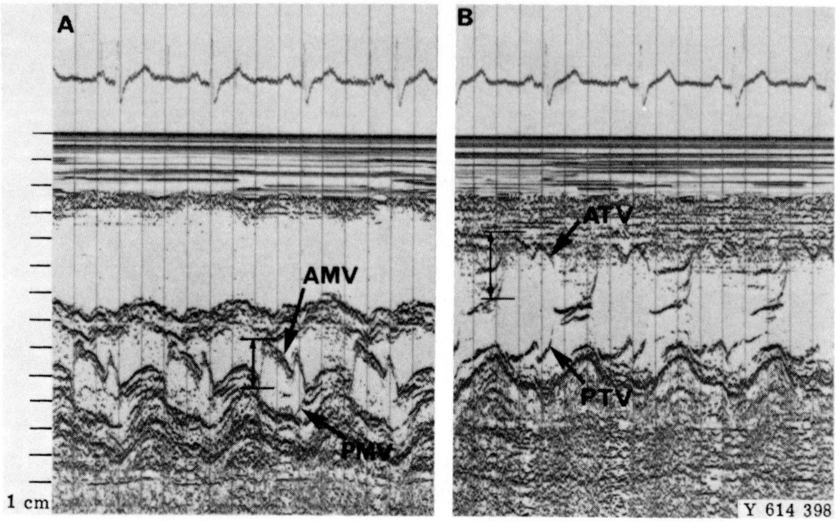

Figure 42. *A*, Patient, age 48, with previously undiagnosed atrial septal defect. Systolic bulging of mitral valve does not approximate septum. Septum appears to come in contact with anterior mitral leaflet in early diastole, probably owing to dilatation of right ventricle; *B*, tricuspid valve from same patient as in *A*. Note increased opening amplitude of anterior tricuspid leaflet compared to opening amplitude of anterior mitral leaflet. This is observed in patients with right ventricular volume overloads and indicates increased blood flow through tricuspid valve. AMV=anterior mitral valve, PMV=posterior mitral valve, ATV=anterior tricuspid valve and PTV=posterior tricuspid valve.

Suggested Reading

Mitral Valve

Bergeron, G., *et al.*: Echocardiographic analysis of mitral valve motion after acute myocardial infarction. Circulation *51*:82, 1975.

Bodenheimer, M., Kotler, M., and Tabatznik, B.: Echocardiography of the mitral valve. Md. State Med. J., *20*:50, 1971.

Chakorn, S., *et al.*: Study of normal and abnormal movements of mitral valve ring using reflected ultrasound. Br. Heart J., *34*:480, 1972.

Dale, G., *et al.*: Different incidences of echographic investigation of the mitral apparatus. J. Radiol. Electrol. Med. Nucl., *54*:189, 1973.

Derman, U.: Changes of the mitral echocardiogram with aging and the influence of atherosclerotic risk factors. Atherosclerosis, *15*:349, 1972.

Dillon, J., *et al.*: Echocardiographic manifestations of valvular vegetations. Am. Heart J., *86*:698, 1973.

Glaser, J., *et al.*: Echocardiographic studies of mitral valve. Am. Heart J., *86*:847, 1973 (letter).

Goodman, D., Harrison, D., and Popp, R.: Echocardiographic features of primary pulmonary hypertension. Am. Heart J., *86*:847, 1973.

Goodman, D., Harrison, D., and Popp, R.: Echocardiographic features of primary pulmonary hypertension. Am. J. Cardiol., *33*:438, 1974.

Johnson, M., *et al.*: Usefulness of echocardiography in patients undergoing mitral valve surgery. J. Thorac. Cardiovasc. Surg., *64*:922, 1972.

Kamigaki, M., and Goldschlager, N.: Echocardiographic analysis of mitral valve motion in atrial septal defect. Am. J. Cardiol., *30*:343, 1972.
Kaye, H.: Problems with the papillary muscles. Br. Med. J., *1*:327, 1974 (letter).
Konecke, L., *et al.*: Abnormal mitral valve motion in patients with elevated left ventricular diastolic pressures. Circulation, *47*:989, 1973.
Laniado, S., *et al.*: A study of the dynamic relations between the mitral valve echogram and phasic mitral flow. Circulation, *51*:104, 1975.
Parisi, A., and Milton, B.: Relation of mitral valve closure to the first heart sound in man: Echocardiographic and phonocardiographic assessment. Am. J. Cardiol., *32*:779, 1973.
Quinones, M., *et al.*: Reduction in the rate of diastolic descent of the mitral valve echogram in patients with altered left ventricular diastolic pressure-volume relations. Circulation, *49*:246, 1974.
Spangler, R., *et al.*: Echocardiographic demonstration of bacterial vegetations in active infective endocarditis. J. Clin. Ultrasound, *1*:126, 1973.
Wharton, C., and Bescos, L.: Mitral valve movement: A study using an ultrasound technique. Br. Heart J., *32*:344, 1970.
Williams, R., and Rudd, M.: Echocardiographic features of endocardial cushion defects. Circulation, *49*:418, 1974.
Winsberg, F., and Mercer, E.: Echocardiography in combined valve disease. Radiology, *105*:405, 1972.
Ziady, G., *et al.*: Diastolic closure rate of mitral valve as determined by ultrasound. Br. Heart J., *35*:560, 1973.

Mitral Valve—Arrhythmia

Chandraratna, P., *et al.*: Abnormal mitral valve motion during ventricular extrasystoles: An echocardiographic study. Am. J. Cardiol., *34*:783, 1974.
DeMaria, A., *et al.*: Echographic assessment of atrial transport, mitral movement, and ventricular performance following electroversion of supraventricular arrhythmias. Circulation, *51*:273, 1975.
Gabor, G., and Winsberg, F.: Motion of mitral valves in cardiac arrhythmias: Ultrasonic cardiographic study. Invest. Radiol., *5*:355, 1970.

Mitral Valve in Aortic Disease

Botvinick, E., *et al.*: Echocardiographic demonstration of early mitral valve closure in severe aortic insufficiency. Its clinical implications, Circulation, *51*:836, 1975.
Craige, E., and Fortuin, J.: Studies on mitral valve motion in the presence of the Austin-Flint murmur. Trans. Am. Clin. Climatol. Assoc., *83*:209, 1972.
Pridie, R. B., Beham, R., and Oakley, C. M.: Echocardiography of the mitral valve in aortic valve disease. Br. Heart J., *33*:296, 1971.
Winsberg, F., Gabor, G., and Hernberg, J.: Fluttering of the mitral valve in aortic insufficiency. Circulation, *41*:225, 1970.

Mitral Valve in IHSS

Abbasi, A., *et al.*: Echocardiographic diagnosis of idiopathic hypertrophic cardiomyopathy without outflow obstruction. Circulation, *46*:897, 1972.
Aigner, A., *et al.*: Asymmetric septal hypertrophy. Ann. Intern. Med., *81*:650, 1974.
Bloom, K., *et al.*: The association of fixed and dynamic left ventricular outflow obstruction. Am. Heart J., *89*:586, 1975.
Bolton, M., Jr., *et al.*: The effects of operation on the echocardiographic features of idiopathic hypertrophic subaortic stenosis. Circulation, *50*:897, 1974.
Chung, K., Manning, J., and Gramiak, R.: Echocardiography in coexisting hypertrophic subaortic stenosis and fixed left ventricular outflow obstruction. Circulation, *49*:673, 1974.
DeLaCalzada, C., *et al.*: Proceedings: Echocardiographic features of hypertrophic obstructive cardiomyopathy. Br. Heart J., *36*:396, 1974.

Hardarson, T., and Curiel, R.: Study of clinical pharmacology of hypertrophic obstructive cardiomyopathy by noninvasive diagnostic investigations. Br. Heart J., *35*:865, 1973.

Henry, W., Clark, C., and Epstein, S.: Asymmetric septal hypertrophy: The unifying link in the IHSS disease spectrum. Observations regarding its pathogenesis, pathophysiology and course. Circulation, *47*:827, 1973.

Henry, W., *et al.*: Echocardiographic measurement of the left ventricular outflow gradient in idiopathic hypertrophic subaortic stenosis. N. Engl. J. Med., *288*:19, 1973.

Johnson, A., Lonky, S., and Carleton, R.: Combined hypertrophic subaortic stenosis and calcific aortic valvular stenosis. Am. J. Cardiol., *35*:706, 1975.

King, J., *et al.*: Markedly abnormal mitral valve motion without simultaneous interventricular pressure gradient due to uneven mitral-septal contact in idiopathic hypertrophic subaortic stenosis. Am. J. Cardiol., *34*:360, 1974.

King, J., *et al.*: Echocardiographic assessment of idiopathic hypertrophic subaortic stenosis. Chest, *64*:723, 1973.

Kossowsky, W., Mohr, B., and Dardashti, I.: Acute myocardial infarction in idiopathic hypertrophic subaortic stenosis. Chest, *64*:529, 1973.

Marcus, G., Popp, R., and Stinson, E.: Coronary-artery disease with IHSS. Lancet, *1*:901, 1974.

Nanda, N., *et al.*: Echocardiography in the diagnosis of idiopathic hypertrophic subaortic stenosis coexisting with aortic valve disease. Circulation, *50*:752, 1974.

Pridie, R., and Oakley, C.: Mechanism of mitral regurgitation in hypertrophic obstructive cardiomyopathy. Br. Heart J., *32*:203, 1970.

Rossen, R., *et al.*: Echocardiographic criteria in the diagnosis of idiopathic hypertrophic subaortic stenosis. Circulation, *50*:747, 1974.

Shah, P.: IHSS—HOCM—MSS—ASH? Circulation, *51*:577, 1975 (editorial).

Shah, P., *et al.*: Role of echocardiography in diagnostic and hemodynamic assessment of hypertrophic subaortic stenosis. Circulation, *44*:891, 1971.

Shah, P., *et al.*: Echocardiographic assessment of the effects of surgery and propranolol on the dynamics of outflow obstruction and hyperpranolol on the dynamics of outflow obstruction and hypertrophic subaortic stenosis. Circulation, *45*:516, 1972.

Tajik, A., and Giuliani, E.: Echocardiographic observations in idiopathic hypertrophic subaortic stenosis. Mayo Clin. Proc., *49*:89, 1974.

Mitral Valve and Left Atrial Masses

Bass, N., and Sharratt, G.: Left atrial myxoma diagnosed by echocardiography, with observations on tumor movement. Br. Heart J., *35*:1332, 1973.

Bodenheimer, M., *et al.*: Echocardiographic features of experimental left atrial tumor. Am. Heart J., *88*:615, 1974.

Croxson, F., *et al.*: Long-term follow-up of atrial myxoma. Br. Heart J., *34*:1018, 1972.

Dodd, M., and Wilcken, D.: Echocardiography in left atrial myxoma: Relation to the findings in mitral stenosis. Aust. N.Z. J. Med., *2*:124, 1972.

Edmands, R. E., *et al.*: Atrial myxoma: A curable disorder. A case report. J. Indiana State Med. Assoc., *67*:903, 1974.

Farooki, Z., *et al.*: Ultrasonic pattern of ventricular rhabdomyoma in two infants. Am. J. Cardiol., *34*:842, 1974.

Feigenbaum, H.: Echocardiography. Philadelphia, Lea & Febiger, p. 152, 1972.

Finegan, R., and Harrison, D.: Diagnosis of left atrial myxoma by echocardiography. N. Engl. J. Med., *282*:1022, 1970.

Gustafson, A., *et al.*: Left atrial myxoma diagnosed by ultrasound cardiography. Angiology, *24*:554, 1973.

Jenzer, H., Follath, F., and Zutter, W.: The echocardiographic diagnosis of atrial myxoma. Schweiz. Med. Wochenschr., *104*:1570, 1974.

Johnson, M., *et al.*: Echocardiographic diagnosis of a left atrial myxoma found attached to the free left atrial wall. J. Clin. Ultrasound, *1*:75, 1973.

Kerber, R., Kelly, D., Jr., and Gutenkauf, C.: Left atrial myxoma. Demonstrated by stop-action cardiac ultrasonography. Am. J. Cardiol., *34*:838, 1974.

Klepacki, Z., Surlowica-Sidun, B., and Zarebska, L.: Intra-atrial thrombus detected by ultrasonocardiography. Kardiol. Pol., *17*:83, 1974.

Kortis, J., and Moghadam, A.: Echocardiographic diagnosis of left atrial myxoma. Chest, *58*:550, 1970.
Lortscher, R., *et al.*: Left atrial myxoma presenting as rheumatic fever. Chest, *66*:302, 1974.
Martinez, E., Giles, T., and Burch, G.: Echocardiographic diagnosis of left atrial myxoma. Am. J. Cardiol., *33*:281, 1974.
Mispireta, L., *et al.*: Tumors of the heart. Med. Ann. DC., *43*:245, 1974.
Moscovitz, H., *et al.*: Simulated left atrial tumor. A hemodynamic, echocardiographic and cineangiographic study. Am. J. Cardiol., *34*:63, 1974.
Nasser, W., *et al.*: Atrial myxoma. Part I: Clinical and pathologic features in nine cases. Am. Heart J., *83*:694, 1972.
Nasser, W., *et al.*: Atrial myxoma. Part II: Phonocardiographic, echocardiographic, hemodynamic and angiographic features in nine cases. Am. Heart J., *83*:810, 1972.
Peters, M., *et al.*: The clinical syndrome of atrial myxoma. JAMA, *230*:695, 1974.
Poehlmann, H., Basta, L., and Brown, R.: Left atrial thrombus detected by ultrasound—a case report. J. Clin. Ultrasound, *3*:65, 1975.
Popp, R., and Levine, R.: Left atrial mass simulating cardiomyopathy. J. Clin. Ultrasound, *1*:96, 1973.
Rees, J., Ross, R., and Keen, G.: Lentiginosis and left atrial myxoma. Br. Heart J., *35*:874, 1973.
Spangler, R., and Okin, T.: Echocardiographic demonstration of left atrial thrombus. Chest, *67*:716, 1975.
Srivastava, T., and Fletecher, E.: The echocardiogram in left atrial myxoma. Am. J. Med., *54*:136, 1973.
Steinmetz, E., Calanchini, P., and Anguilar, M.: Left atrial myxoma as a neurological problem: A case report and review. Stroke, *4*:451, 1973.
Sung, R., *et al.*: Hemodynamic features of prolapsing and non-prolapsing left atrial myxoma. Circulation, *51*:342, 1975.
Tallury, V., and DePasquale, N.: Ultrasound cardiography in the diagnosis of left atrial thrombosis. Chest, *59*:501, 1971.
Zackia, A., *et al.*: Recurrence of left atrial myxoma. J. Cardiovasc. Surg. (Torino), *25*:467, 1974.

Mitral Valve with Mitral Disease

Burgess, J., *et al.*: Echocardiographic findings in different types of mitral regurgitation. Circulation, *48*:97, 1973.
Duchak, J., Jr., *et al.*: The posterior mitral valve echo and the echocardiographic diagnosis of mitral stenosis. Am. J. Cardiol., *29*:628, 1972.
Flaherty, J., Livengood, S., and Fortuin, N.: Atypical posterior leaflet motion in echocardiogram in mitral stenosis. Am. J. Cardiol., *35*:675, 1975.
Fortuin, N., and Craige, E.: Echocardiographic studies of genesis of mitral diastolic murmurs. Br. Heart J., *35*:75, 1973.
Freeman, J., Hitt, J., and Rinaldo, J.: Mitral leaflet velocity in the determination of mitral stenosis. Med. Res. Eng., *11*:4, 1972.
Giles, T., Burch, G., and Martinez, E.: Value of exploratory "scanning" in the echocardiographic diagnosis of ruptured chordae tendineae. Circulation, *49*:678, 1974.
Levisman, J., Abbasi, A., and Pearce, M.: Posterior mitral leaflet motion in mitral stenosis. Circulation, *51*:511, 1975.
Lundstrom, N.: Echocardiograph in the diagnosis of congenital mitral stenosis and an evaluation of the results of mitral valvulotomy. Circulation, *46*:44, 1972.
McLaurin, L., *et al.*: An appraisal of mitral valve echocardiograms mimicking mitral stenosis in conditions with right ventricular pressure overload. Circulation, *48*:801, 1973.
Madeira, H., *et al.*: Echocardiographic assessment of left ventricular volume overload. Br. Heart J., *36*:1175, 1974.
Mary, D., *et al.*: Study with reflected ultrasound of patients with mitral valve repair. Br. Heart J., *35*:480, 1973.

Millward, D., McLaurin, L., and Craige, E.: Echocardiographic studies to explain opening snaps in presence of non-stenotic mitral valves. Am. J. Cardiol., *31*:64, 1973.

Millward, D., McLaurin, L., and Craige, E.: Echocardiographic studies of the mitral valve in patients with congestive cardiomyopathy and mitral regurgitation. Am. Heart J., *85*:413, 1973.

Nanda, N., *et al.*: Mitral commissurotomy versus replacement: Preoperative evaluation by echocardiography. Circulation, *51*:263, 1975.

Rothbaum, D., DeJoseph, R., and Tavel, M.: Diastolic heart sound produced by mid-diastolic closure of the mitral valve. Am. J. Cardiol., *34*:367, 1974.

Rubenstein, J., *et al.*: The echocardiographic determination of mitral valve opening and closure: Correlation with hemodynamic studies in man. Circulation, *51*:98, 1975.

Silver, W., Rodriquez-Torres, R., and Newfelt, E.: The echocardiogram in a case of mitral stenosis before and after surgery. Am. Heart J., *78*:811, 1969.

Sweatman, T., Selzer, A., and Cohn, K.: Echocardiographic diagnosis of ruptured chordae tendineae. Am. J. Cardiol., *26*:661, 1970.

Sweatman, T., *et al.*: Echocardiographic diagnosis of mitral regurgitation due to ruptured chordae tendineae. Circulation, *46*:580, 1972.

Yuste, P., *et al.*: Ultrasonic analysis of mitral stenosis: pre and post operative studies. Rev. Esp. Cardiol., *26*:85, 1973.

Mitral Valve—Prolapsing

DeMaria, A., *et al.*: The variable spectrum of echocardiographic manifestations of the mitral valve prolapse syndrome. Circulation, *50*:33, 1974.

Dillon, J., *et al.*: Use of echocardiography in patients with prolapsed mitral valve. Circulation, *43*:503, 1971.

Goodman, D., Shappell, S., and Brown, R.: Echocardiogram of mitral valve prolapse. Circulation, *49*:780, 1974 (letter).

LeWinter, M., *et al.*: Phenylephrine-induced atypical chest pain in patients with prolapsing mitral valve leaflets. Am. J., Cardiol., *34*:12, 1974.

Luisada, A., and Bhat, P.: Systolic click and late systolic murmur in a young woman. Chest, *66*:292, 1974.

Popp, R., *et al.*: Echocardiographic abnormalities in the mitral valve prolapse syndrome. Circulation, *49*:428, 1974.

Shappell, S., *et al.*: Sudden death and the familial occurrence of mid-systolic click, late systolic murmur syndrome. Circulation, *48*:1128, 1973.

Winkle, R., Goodman, D., and Popp, R.: Simultaneous echocardiographic-phonocardiographic recordings at rest and during amyl nitrite administration in patients with mitral valve prolapse. Circulation, *51*:522, 1975.

4

LEFT ATRIUM, AORTA AND AORTIC VALVE

Left Atrium and Aorta

The lower left atrial wall begins at the junction where the ultrasound beam leaves the left ventricle and the posterior mitral leaflet drops out of the tracing (Figure 43).

The motion of the left atrial wall should not be confused with the motion of the left ventricular wall at any time. If one examines the electrocardiogram with the echocardiogram, the left atrial wall is seen to move away from the transducer with the onset of systole; with the onset of diastole the wall moves abruptly forward toward the transducer. This is exactly opposite to the motion of the left ventricular wall.

The septum is seen to attenuate and gradually become the anterior aortic wall as the transducer is angled superiorly from the mitral valve and rotated medially toward the right shoulder. If the transducer is scanned higher into the left atrium to the point where the aortic valve is seen, the motion of the left atrial wall diminishes. Often there is a second line above or below what is supposed to be the left atrial wall, confusing the interpretation of where the proper dimension should be taken (Figure 43, arrow). It is very possible for both lines to represent the left atrial wall, since this chamber is a curved structure. The lateral beam width may be picking up portions of the curvature of the left atrial wall which will be graphically recorded as multiple moving lines. To be consistent in our measurements, we scan the area between the mitral valve and the high left atrium and aortic valve several times to

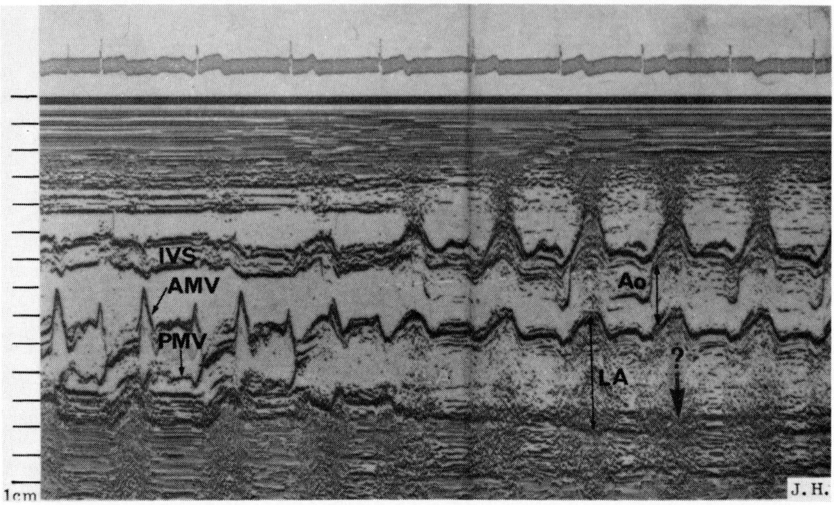

Figure 43. Scan from mitral valve to left atrium and aorta. IVS = interventricular septum, AMV = anterior mitral valve, PMV = posterior mitral valve, Ao = aorta, LA = left atrium and large arrow = possible left atrial wall moving into sound beam simultaneously with that portion of left atrial wall used to measure standard left atrial dimension.

ascertain which wall is the most dominant and possesses the most continuity.

Figure 44 is a scan from the aortic valve to the mitral valve. There is another line below the posterior aortic wall (Figure 44). The origin of the structure has not been established. To be consistent about measuring the left atrium, this secondary line should be ignored and the aortic wall with the most continuity with the mitral valve should be measured.

Many examiners have difficulty in trying to record a good aortic valve tracing. The reason for this is that the transducer was scanned to the area of the aortic outflow tract and then stopped rather than being angled more superiorly and medially toward the right shoulder. If the heart is positioned vertically within the chest, the transducer must be tilted more superiorly than usual; if it is positioned horizontally, as in short, obese patients, the transducer must be tilted more medially to obtain the aortic leaflets and the passive portion of the posterior left atrial wall.

Aortic Root Aneurysms

Aortic root aneurysms are found in the area where the aortic valve is seated and slightly above the location of aortic leaflets. The transducer must be angled higher beyond the aortic valve. If an aneurysm is present, the aorta should suddenly become considerably wider (Figure 45).

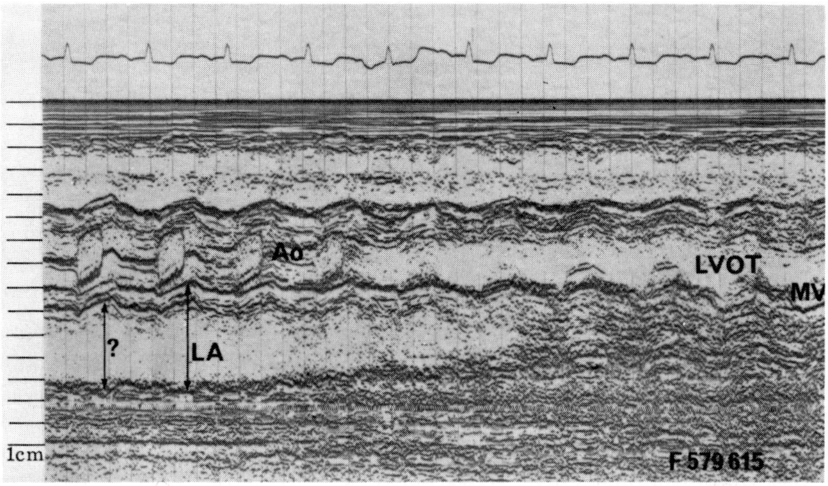

Figure 44. Scan from aortic to mitral valve in technically difficult patient. Origin of secondary line with no continuity with mitral valve may be anterior left atrial wall, but this is pure speculation. Ao = aorta, LA = left atrium, LVOT = left ventricular outflow tract and MV = mitral valve.

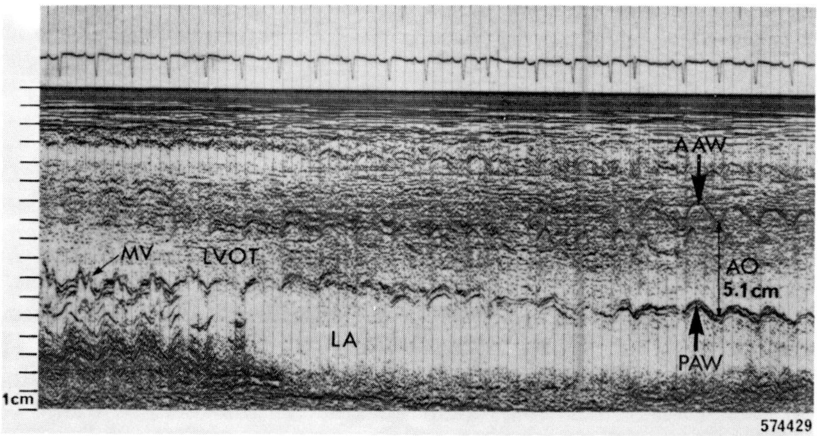

Figure 45. Scan from mitral valve to position above aortic valve. Ordinarily aortic dimension widens only slightly as beam becomes more oblique to aortic vessel. Sudden widening should cause suspicion of aortic aneurysm. MV = mitral valve, LVOT = left ventricular outflow tract, LA = left atrium, AAW = anterior aortic wall, PAW = posterior aortic wall and AO = aorta.

Left Atrial Clot

One of the most hazardous diagnoses to make is identification of left atrial clot. So far we have either made only tentative guesses before catheterization or tried to determine a large mural clot on the echogram after it was discovered during mitral valve replacement procedures.

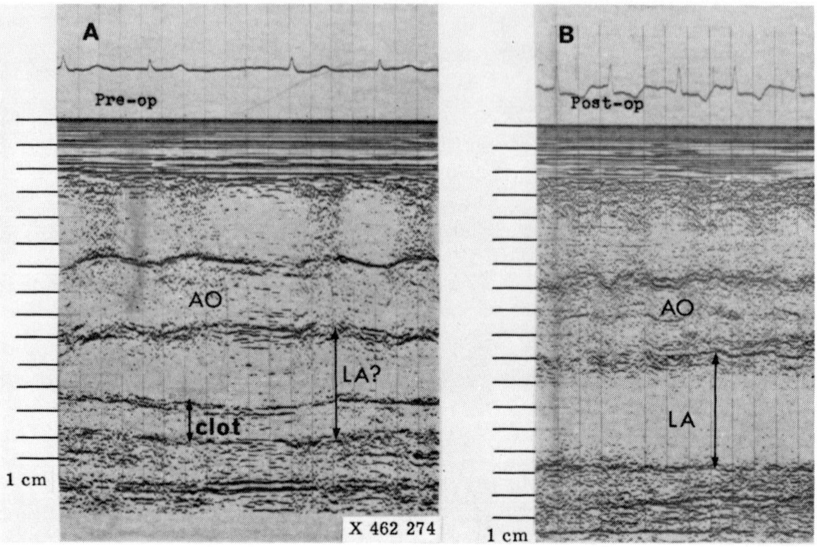

Figure 46. *A*, Preoperative tracing from patient with calcific mitral stenosis and mild mitral insufficiency. Atrial appendage did not fill during cineangiography; *B*, postoperative left atrial tracing. "Clot" echo could not be found. AO = aorta and LA = left atrium.

Figure 46 is from a patient who had a very large mural clot identified during surgical procedure. As nearly as could be managed, the plane of the ultrasound beam was identical in both examinations. The only difference in the two tracings is an additional strong echo anterior to the left atrial wall which was identified by scanning to the mitral valve. There appears to be an echo-free space between the leading edge of the "clot" and the left atrial wall, as would be expected from homogeneous material (Figure 46*A*). Postoperatively this strong echo was absent.

Free-floating left atrial clot is not common. Figure 47 represents the first clot of this type seen at this laboratory, and it was not identified until performance of cineangiography. Since the identification of this clot in 1972, two others have been seen and identified prior to invasive procedures preceding surgical intervention.

This patient's catheterization data disclosed moderately severe mitral stenosis with a very large left atrium and a clot in the atrial appendage. There was also thought to be a mobile clot within the body of the left atrium. Mild mitral insufficiency was present. Owing to exacerbation of the mitral stenosis (MVA = 1.3 cm^2 from 2.1 cm^2) and deterioration of the patient, surgical treatment was recommended.

During the operative procedure the surgeon found: ". . . a free floating tumor mass in the left atrium. This measured about two by 4 centimeters. No stalk was apparent and no site of attachment could be

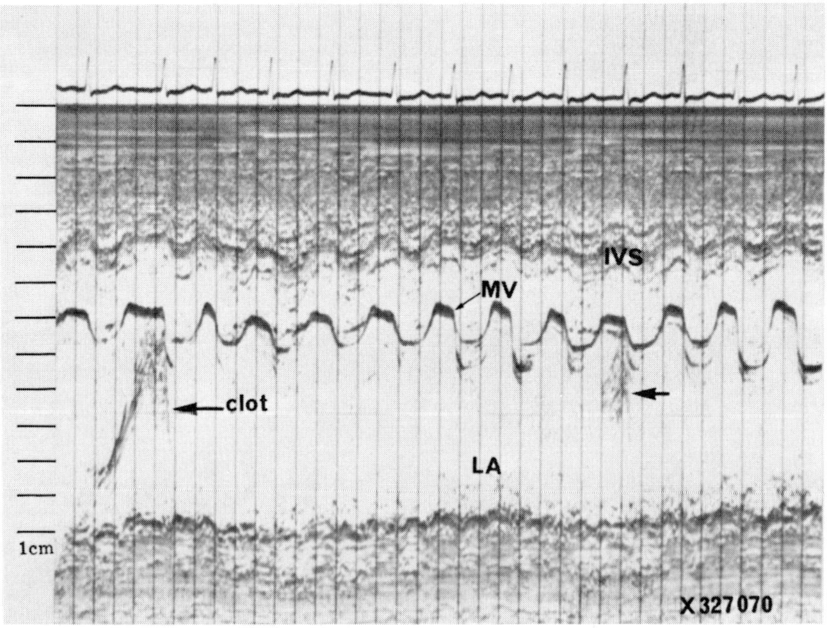

Figure 47. Free-floating left atrial thrombus prevented from entering mitral orifice by obstruction of mitral stenosis. Transducer was angled toward left ventricular outflow tract and held motionless. Clot periodically passed in and out of sound beam as it moved around within left atrium. MV = mitral valve, IVS = interventricular septum and LA = left atrium.

seen on the left atrial wall. This tumor mass was presumed to be a thrombus that either had arisen spontaneously in the large fibrillating atrium or had originally been attached to the left atrial wall and then later became free. No other left atrial clot was present."

Aortic Valve

Normal Aortic Valve

The normal aortic valve appears as a parallelogram with thin and widely opening cusps (Figure 48). The right aortic leaflet or more commonly, anterior aortic leaflet, opens toward the transducer with the onset of systole. The posterior aortic cusp opens away from the transducer with the onset of systole. The two leaflets remain widely apart during systole and then close together to meet when systole is completed.

The aortic lumen containing the leaflets is free of heavy and multiple echoes, and the aortic walls move well in response to the vigorous systolic contraction and the force of blood entering the aorta.

The cusps' separation may be measured as the leaflets initially reach their maximum separation, or they may be measured during

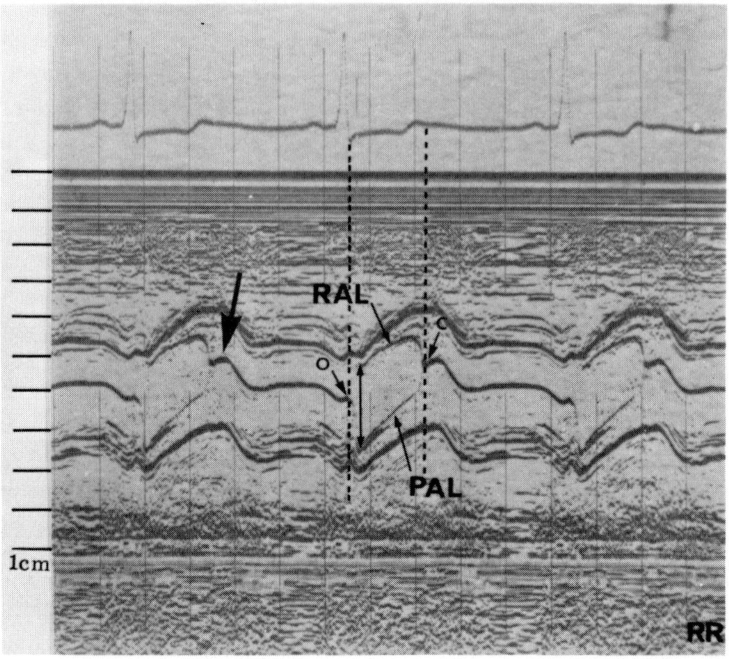

Figure 48. Normal aortic valve within normal aortic root. RAL = right (or anterior) aortic leaflet, PAL = posterior aortic leaflet, o = initial opening of the valve, c = closure of the valve and unmarked arrow = normal anterior motion.

midsystole. However, the cusps' separation should not be measured during late systole since the volume of blood flow through the cusps is beginning to diminish and the cusps tend to float toward a closed position.

The anterior "humping" of the aortic valve following closure of the valve is a common occurrence in patients with efficient cardiac outputs. It may be a total displacement of the aortic root anteriorly following systole's completion and does not seem to indicate abnormality.

Aortic Valve with Aortic Insufficiency

In aortic insufficiency the valve may often appear to be normal even though the valve is significantly diseased. The cusps may appear thin and may open wider than normal, especially if the aortic root is dilated, and the cusps may coapt properly during diastole. The cusps may appear to open eccentrically within the aortic root, but one should be careful in calling an aortic valve bicuspid on the basis of eccentricity of valve opening. As will be discussed, recording technique can cause the valve to open eccentrically.

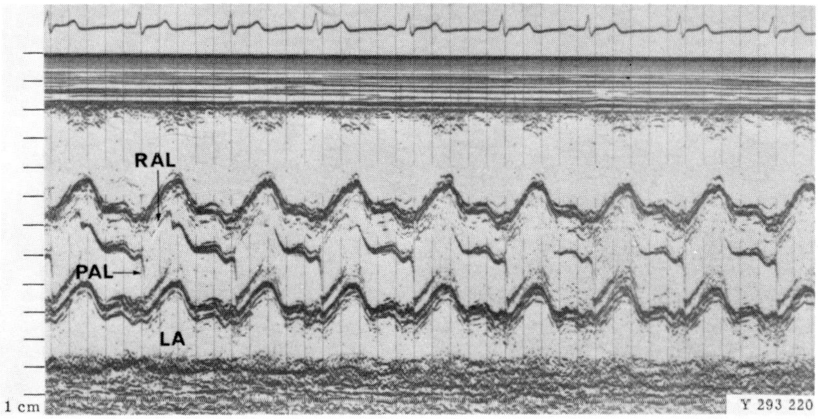

Figure 49. Aortic valve from patient with aortic insufficiency. Posterior leaflet has more opening amplitude than has anterior leaflet, but this may be owing to position from which valve was recorded. RAL = right aortic leaflet, PAL = posterior aortic leaflet and LA = left atrium.

Figure 49 is from a patient with aortic insufficiency secondary to rheumatic heart disease. The leaflets are not remarkable except for some eccentricity of opening. Aortic insufficiency is not evident on the aortic valve tracing. The diagnosis was determined from fluttering of the mitral valve and dilatation of the left ventricle.

As the aortic valve becomes diseased, the leaflets begin to thicken and a multiplicity of echoes are seen within the aortic lumen. The cusps' separation is neither easily visualized nor interpreted. In fact the measurements derived from the cusps' separation may be totally erroneous, as seen from the valve opening in Figure 50, complexes 1, 2 and 3. Trying to determine which cusps' separation is the right one is difficult and should be approached with caution.

The patient described in Figure 50 came to catheterization for evaluation of mitral stenosis. She had pulmonary hypertension, severe mitral stenosis and minimal aortic insufficiency. The cardiac output measured 4.3 L/min with a cardiac index of 2.8 L/min/M^2. No aortic gradient was measured across the valve.

Aortic Valve with Aortic Stenosis

A severely stenosed aortic valve may show an aortic lumen almost completely filled with echoes. The leaflets become very difficult to identify, and the cusps' separation is poorly, if at all, visualized. The valve is so distorted, in fact, that the cusps' separation should not be measured.

The more severe the aortic stenosis, the more the aortic root becomes ectatic. The cusps cannot be recorded from the usual position along the left sternal border. Recording leaflet motion will be easier if the

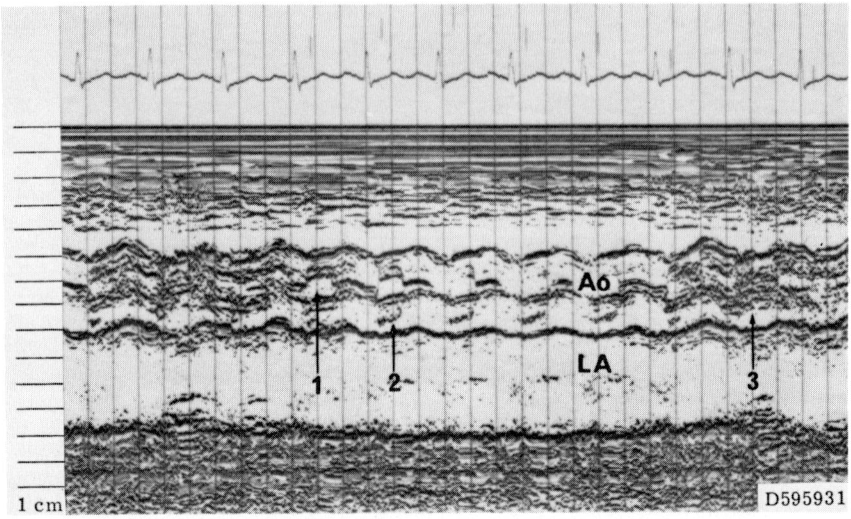

Figure 50. Patient, age 47, with no measurable gradient across aortic valve. Aortic insufficiency was minimal. Tracing demonstrates difficulty in determining which aortic cusp separation is representative of existing orifice. Ao = aorta and LA = left atrium.

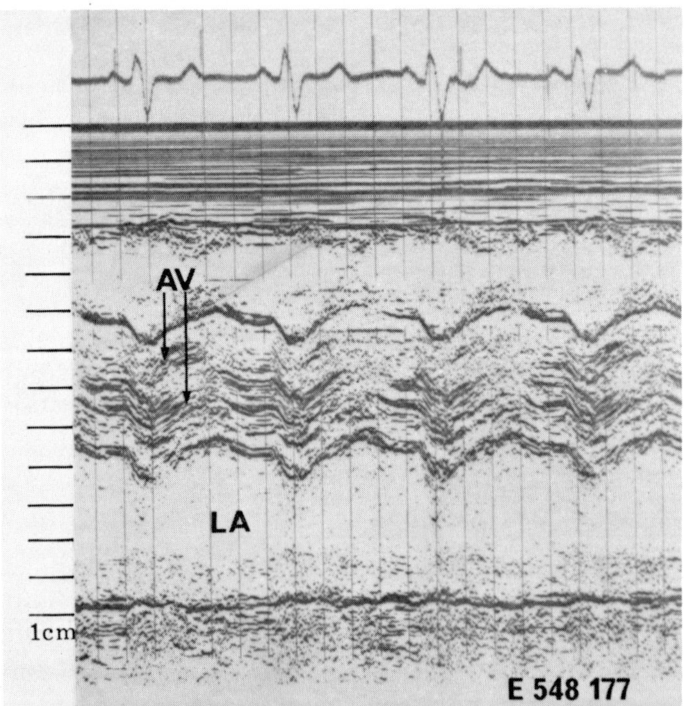

Figure 51. Severe aortic stenosis in 44-year-old man. Valve should be described as thickened with poor cusps' separation. Aortic walls do not appear to be involved; coronary arteries were normal at catheterization. AV = aortic valve and LA = left atrium.

transducer is moved laterally toward the point of maximal impulse at the apex and angled in a plane with the long axis of the heart. The left atrial dimension will probably be distorted from this position and can be ignored.

Figure 51 is a tracing from a patient with catheterization-proven aortic stenosis. The aortic gradient measured 110 mm Hg with moderate aortic insufficiency; cardiac output was 4.4 L/min with a cardiac index of 2.3 L/min/M^2. The valve was described at operation as being heavily calcified with stenotic funnel-shaped aortic cusps.

The amount of aortic gradient across the valve cannot be estimated by the appearance of the cusps on the echocardiogram. The patient of Figure 52 was brought to catheterization, at which time a 39 mm Hg gradient at rest was measured across the aortic valve. Cardiac output was 3.0 L/min with a cardiac index of 1.7 L/min/M^2. Severe aortic insufficiency was seen with cineangiography. Moderate mitral stenosis was also present.

In contrast, Figure 53 was taken from a patient with a 30 mm Hg gradient across the aortic valve. Cardiac output was 5.5 L/min with a cardiac index of 2.9 L/min/M^2. In addition severe triple-vessel coronary artery disease was discovered.

Although one would be tempted to measure the amount of cusps' separation in Figure 52, the urge should be resisted. Although the

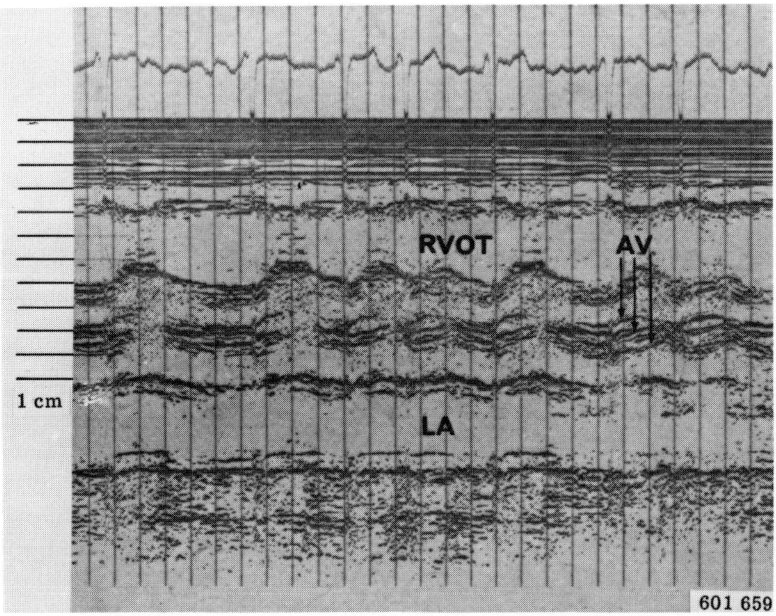

Figure 52. Patient, age 55, with severe aortic valve disease and mitral stenosis. Aortic cusps' separation should not be measured. RVOT = right ventricular outflow tract, AV = aortic valve and LA = left atrium.

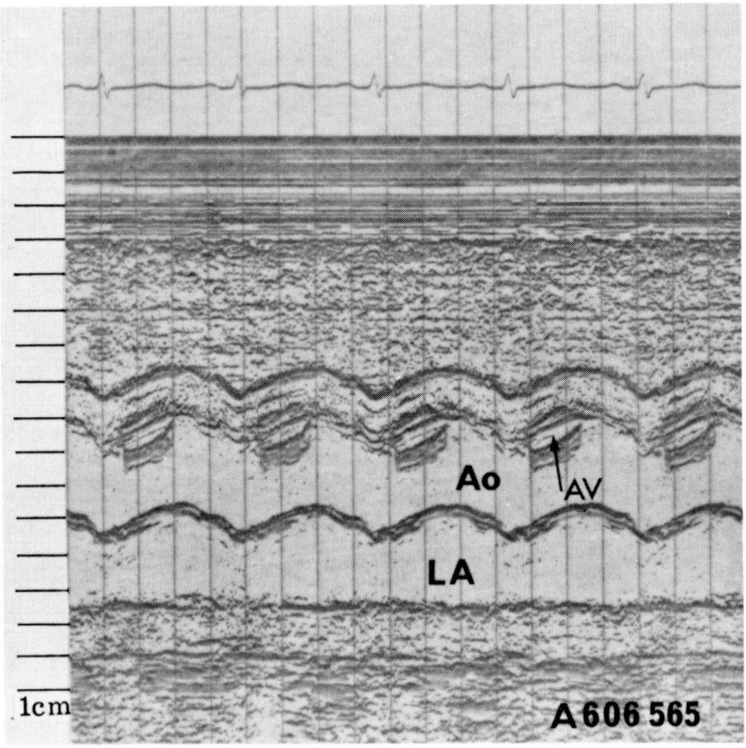

Figure 53. Patient, age 58, with mild to moderate calcific aortic valvular disease and severe ischemic heart disease. Ao = aorta, LA = left atrium and AV = aortic valve.

cusps' separation appears similar to that seen in Figure 53, the degree of aortic stenosis is not similar. One can probably do well separating the mild aortic from the severe aortic stenosis by echocardiography, but the wide range of moderate aortic stenosis may be badly interpreted if one tries to quantify it.

Figure 54 is a tracing from a patient with a thickened aortic valve, which appears similar to Figure 51. The anterior aortic cusp appears to be thick and immobile. The posterior cusp is thickened but more mobile, contributing most to the apparent orifice. At catheterization the patient demonstrated a 65 mm Hg gradient across the aortic valve. Left ventricular pressure was 250/30 mm Hg. Cardiac output was 4.8 L/min. By cineangiography the aortic valve was seen to be competent and heavily calcified. The aortic valve area was calculated to be 0.5 cm^2.

The technique used to record aortic cusps needs to be evaluated continually. Figure 55*A* was recorded just as the transducer was angled superiorly from the mitral valve toward the aorta. However, the

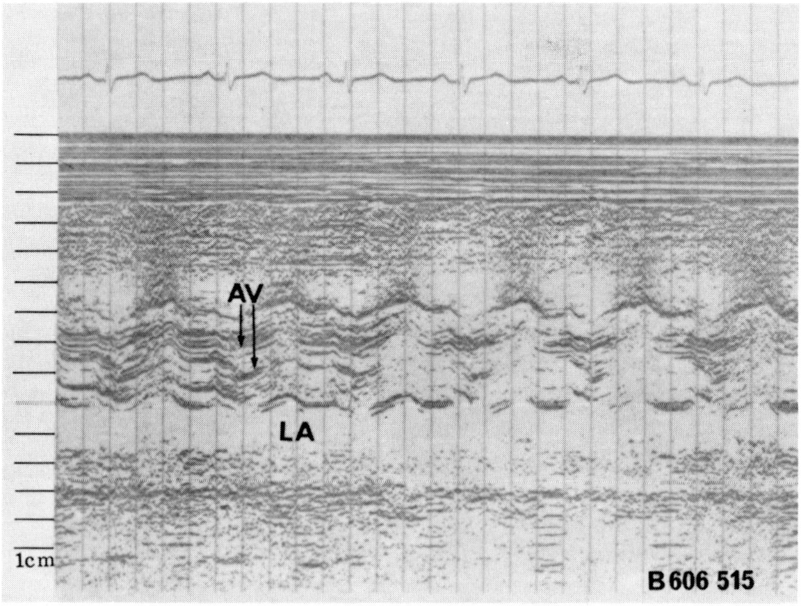

Figure 54. Patient, age 61, with severe aortic stenosis. AV = aortic valve and LA = left atrium.

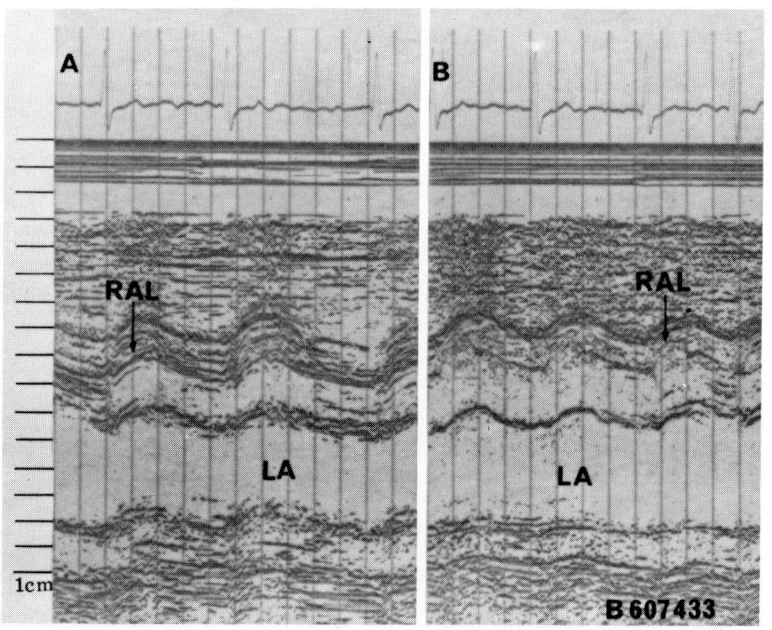

Figure 55. Patient, age 35, evaluated for mitral stenosis. No aortic stenosis was detected by cardiac catheterization. RAL = right (anterior) aortic leaflet and LA = left atrium.

transducer was not angled medially enough, and the aortic valve appears to have a thickened anterior cusp. Figure 55*B* was obtained from the same patient. The transducer was angled properly, and the aortic leaflets are well identified; the cusps are thin and open normally. The right (anterior) cusp no longer appears thickened. Catheterization was performed to evaluate mitral stenosis. No aortic stenosis was demonstrated. Cardiac output was 4.5 L/min with an index of 2.25 L/min/M^2.

Congenital Aortic Stenosis

Diagnosing aortic stenosis in children is misleading by M-mode echocardiography. Figure 56 is from a 4-year-old child with catheterization-proven aortic stenosis. The gradient across the aortic valve was approximately 85 mm Hg.

The cusps appear to open well and do not appear to be thickened. The reason for this finding is that the sound beam is passing through the domed portion of the valve. The site of stenosis is at the top of the dome where the leaflets are fused.

One must be aware that the recorded tracing is not always the correct one. The aortic valve recorded from the fifth intercostal space (Figure 57*A*) shows a thickened valve that does not appear to open well. Figure 57*B* was recorded from the sixth intercostal space in the same patient. Although the anterior cusp is not visualized, the posterior leaflet is seen to open with sufficient amplitude and to exhibit some fluttering, which is normal. The patient was brought to cardiac catheterization to evaluate mitral stenosis and insufficiency. No aortic gradient was

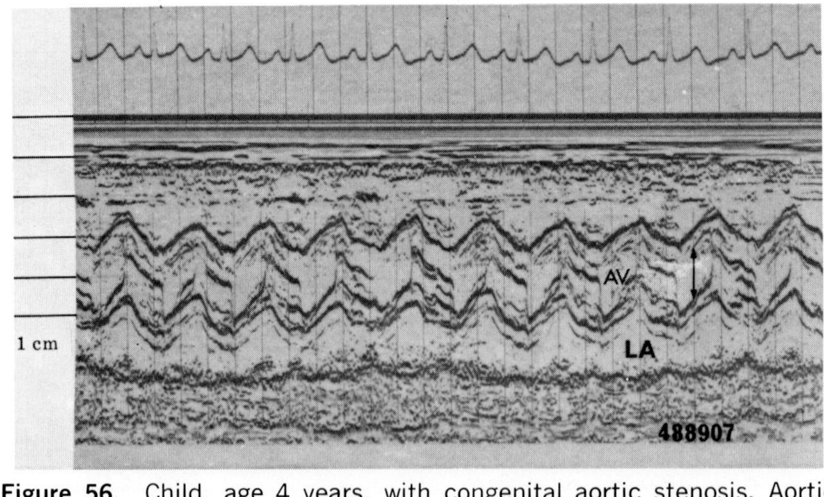

Figure 56. Child, age 4 years, with congenital aortic stenosis. Aortic leaflets appear to open normally as far as aortic wall will allow. Diastolic pattern is unusual in that leaflets do not appear to coapt properly. This feature may be real or artifactual. AV = aortic valve and LA = left atrium.

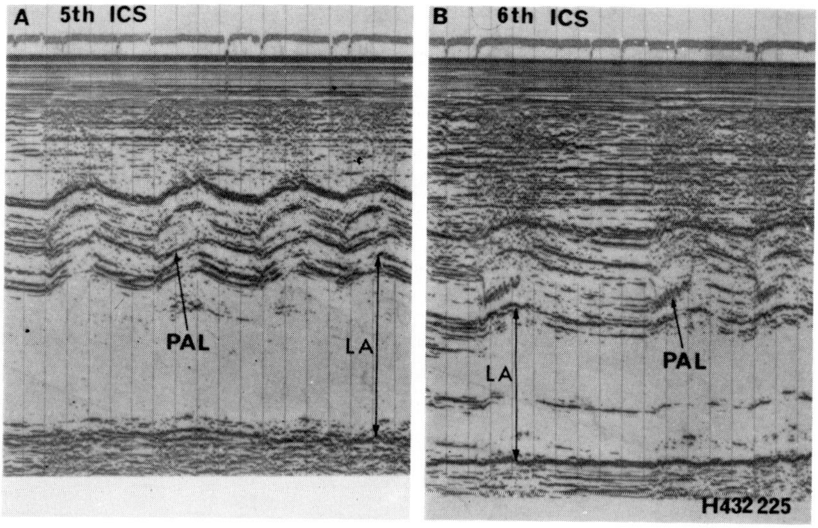

Figure 57. Patient, age 60, with moderate calcific mitral stenosis and mild to moderate mitral insufficiency. Cardiac output was 5.3 L/min with cardiac index of 3.3 L/min/M². Cineangiograms disclosed no restriction or insufficiency of aortic valve. Coronary artery studies were normal. PAL = posterior aortic leaflet and LA = left atrium.

demonstrated across the aortic valve. It is possible that the valve was diseased, but if it was, the lesion was not severe enough either to alter the hemodynamics measured at catheterization or to produce clinical symptoms.

Aortic Valve Motion with Subaortic Obstruction

The aortic valve will respond to diseases that are not directly related to the aortic valve itself. IHSS, *e.g.*, causes the interventricular septum to hypertrophy, and the classic bulging of the mitral valve during systole obstructs the left ventricular outflow tract (Figure 58, unmarked arrow). Discrete subaortic stenosis also causes obstruction of the left ventricular outflow tract but without either hypertrophy of the septum or remarkable systolic bulging of the mitral valve. A diaphragm which is fixed below the aortic valve acts as the obstruction to normal blood flow.

When the left ventricular outflow tract is obstructed, the flow of blood is either reduced or shut off entirely. If no blood passes through the aortic leaflets, the leaflets will close. Rarely do both cusps of the aortic valve close entirely and remain closed from midsystole to the end of systole. Most often either the anterior or the posterior leaflet closes in midsystole in response to the reduced blood flow (Figure 59). As the obstruction below the aortic valve moves away from the septum, blood may continue to pass through the left ventricular outflow tract into the

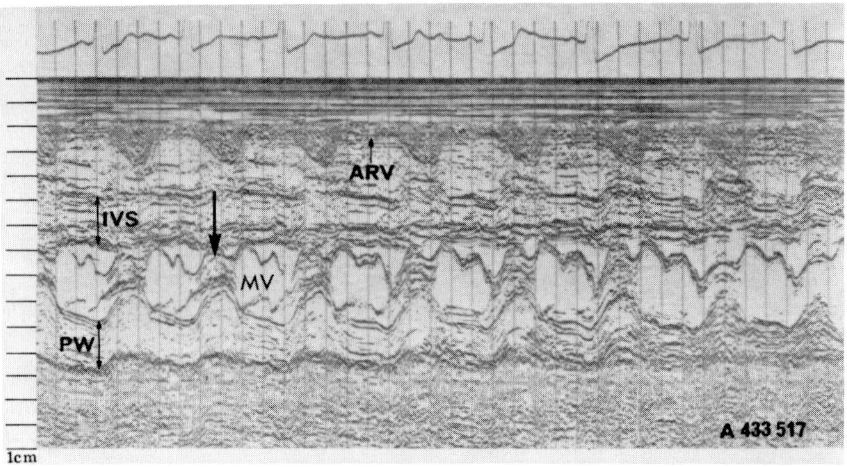

Figure 58. Classic tracing of severe, hypertrophic subaortic stenosis. After long trial of propranolol, patient underwent myomectomy in an attempt to relieve left ventricular outflow obstruction. IVS = interventricular septum, PW = posterior left ventricular wall, MV = mitral valve, ARV = anterior right ventricular wall and unmarked arrow = systolic bulging of mitral valve.

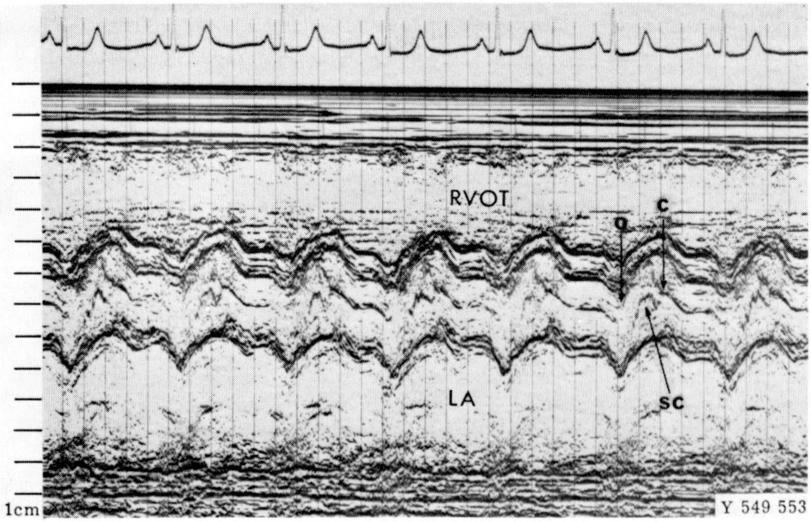

Figure 59. Aortic valve tracing from same patient as in Figure 58. Posterior leaflet of aortic valve closes in midsystole and reopens short time later as mitral valve moves away from left ventricular outflow tract, relieving obstruction to blood flow. RVOT = right ventricular outflow tract, LA = left atrium, o = initial opening of aortic valve, sc = systolic closure and c = closure of aortic valve at end of systole.

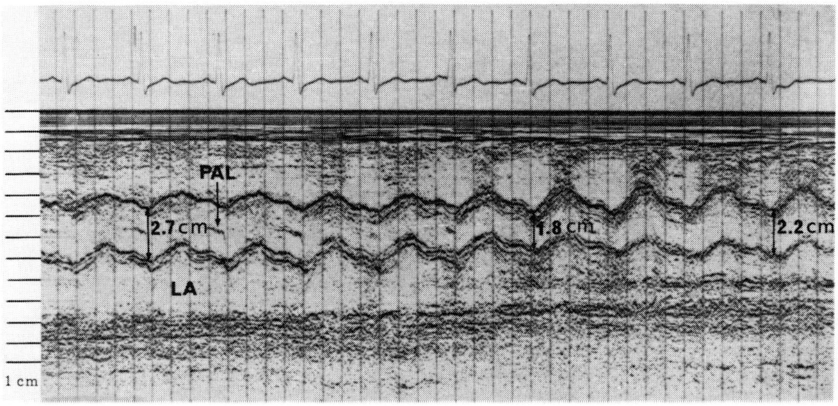

Figure 60. Scan from seat of aortic valve to area above aortic valve, demonstrating moderate supravalvular aortic stenosis. Gradient across obstruction measured 76 mm Hg. Patient was 14 years old. LA = left atrium and PAL = posterior aortic leaflet.

aorta during the latter part of systole; the aortic leaflets reopen, but not as widely as at the onset of systole.

Supravalvular Aortic Stenosis

The most noticeable feature in Figure 60 is the narrowing of the aorta above the seat of the aortic valve. This type of tracing is obtained by tilting the transducer from the area in which aortic leaflets are seen to open and close to the area above the valve and beyond as far as the walls of the aorta are well defined.

Ordinarily as the transducer is tilted above the aortic valve, the dimension of the vessel becomes somewhat wider, because the ultrasonic beam is oblique to the true cross section of the aorta. If the dimension narrows consistently as in Figure 60, supravalvular stenosis is probably present.

Suggested Reading

Left Atrium and Aorta

Brown, O., Harrison, D., and Popp, R.: An improved method for echographic detection of left atrial enlargement. Circulation, *50*:58, 1974.

Chandraratna, P.: Determination of zero reference level for left atrial pressure by echocardiography. Am. Heart J., *89*:159, 1975.

Chandraratna, P., *et al.*: Echocardiographic findings in persistent truncus arteriosus in a young adult. Br. Heart J., *36*:732, 1974.

Chestler, E., *et al.*: Supravalvular stenosing ring of the left atrium associated with corrected transposition of the great vessels. Am. J. Cardiol., *31*:84, 1973.

Chung, K., *et al.*: Isolated supravalvular stenosing ring of left atrium diagnosis before operation and successful surgical treatment. Chest, *65*:25, 1974.

French, J., and Popp, R.: Variability of echocardiographic discontinuity in double outlet right ventricle and truncus arteriosus. Circulation, *51*:848, 1975.

Gibson, D., Honey, M., and Lennox, S.: Cor triatriatum. Diagnosis by echocardiography. Br. Heart J., *36*:835, 1974.
Goldberg, B.: Suprasternal ultrasonography. JAMA, *215*:245, 1971.
Gramiak, R., and Shah, P.: Echocardiography of the aortic root. Invest. Radiol., *3*:356, 1968.
Hirata, T., *et al.*: Estimation of left atrial size using ultrasound. Am. Heart J., *78*:43, 1969.
Kronzon, I., and Mehta, S.: Giant left atrium. Chest, *65*:677, 1974.
Nanda, N., Gramiak, R., and Shah, P.: Diagnosis of aortic root dissection by echocardiography. Circulation, *48*:506, 1973.
Nimura, Y., *et al.*: Non-invasive preoperative diagnosis of cor triatriatum with ultrasonocardiotomogram and conventional echocardiogram. Am. Heart J., *88*:240, 1974.
Sasse, L.: Echocardiography of left atrial wall. JAMA *228*:1667, 1974.
Strunk, B., *et al.*: Echocardiographic recognition of the mitral valve-posterior aortic wall relationship. Circulation, *51*:594, 1975.
TenCate, F., *et al.*: Dimensions and volumes of left atrium and ventricle determined by single beam echocardiography. Br. Heart J., *36*:737, 1974.
Troy, B., *et al.*: Diagnosis of cor-triatriatum by echocardiography. J. Clin. Ultrasound, *1*:257, 1973.
Winsberg, F., and Goldman, H.: Echo patterns of cardiac posterior wall. Invest. Radiol., *4*:173, 1969.

Aortic Valve

Cooperberg, P., *et al.*: Rupture of a sinus Valsalva aneurysm. Report of a case diagnosed preoperatively by echocardiography. Radiology, *113*:171, 1974.
DeMaria, A., *et al.*: Echography and phonography of acute aortic regurgitation in bacterial endocarditis. Ann. Intern. Med., *82*:329, 1975.
Dillon, J., *et al.*: Echocardiographic manifestations of valvular vegetations. Am. Heart J., *86*:698, 1973.
Dillon, J., *et al.*: Echocardiographic manifestations of d-transposition of the great vessels. Am. J. Cardiol., *32*:74, 1973.
Feizi, O., Symons, C., and Yacoub, M.: Echocardiography of normal and diseased aortic valve. Br. Heart J., *35*:560, 1973.
Feizi, O., Symons, C., and Yacoub, M.: Echocardiography of the aortic valve. Studies of normal aortic valve, aortic stenosis, aortic regurgitation and mixed aortic valve disease. Br. Heart J., *36*:341, 1974.
Glaser, J., Whitman, V., and Liebman, J.: Echocardiogram in d-transposition of great vessels. Am. J. Cardiol., *33*:320, 1974 (letter).
Goldberg, B.: Ultrasonic measurement of the aortic arch, right pulmonary artery and left atrium. Radiology, *101*:383, 1971.
Gottlieb, S., *et al.*: Echocardiographic diagnosis of aortic valve vegetations in candida endocarditis. Circulation, *50*:826, 1974.
Gramiak, R., *et al.*: Echocardiographic diagnosis of transposition of the great vessels. Radiology, *106*:187, 1973.
Gramiak, R., and Shah, P.: Echocardiography of the normal and diseased aortic valve. Radiology, *96*:1, 1970.
Hernberg, J., Weiss, B., and Keegan, A.: The ultrasonic recording of aortic valve motion. Radiology, *94*:361, 1970.
Johnson, M., *et al.*: Echocardiography of the aortic valve in non-rheumatic left ventricular outflow tract lesions. Radiology, *112*:677, 1974.
Kelly, D., Wulfsberg, E., and Rowe, R.: Discrete subaortic stenosis. Circulation, *46*:309, 1972.
King, D., Steeg, C., and Ellis, K.: Demonstration of transposition of the great arteries by cardiac ultrasonography. Radiology, *107*:181, 1973.
Kronzon, I., and Mehta, S.: Illustrative echocardiogram: Aortic root dissection. Chest, *65*:88, 1974.
Martinez, E., Burch, G., and Giles, T.: Echocardiographic diagnosis of vegetative aortic bacterial endocarditis. Am. J. Cardiol., *34*:845, 1974.

Millward, D., Robinson, N., and Craige, E.: Dissecting aortic aneurysm diagnosed by echocardiography in a patient with rupture of the aneurysm into the right atrium. Am. J. Cardiol., *30*:427, 1972.

Nanda, N., *et al.*: Echocardiography in the diagnosis of idiopathic hypertrophic subaortic stenosis co-existing with aortic valve disease. Circulation, *50*:752, 1974.

Nanda, N., *et al.*: Echocardiographic recognition of the congenital bicuspid aortic valve. Circulation, *49*:870, 1974.

Nanda, N., *et al.*: Echocardiography of the intra-atrial baffle in dextro-transposition of the great vessels. Circulation, *51*:1130, 1975.

Popp, R., *et al.*: Echocardiographic findings in discrete subvalvular aortic stenosis. Circulation, *49*:226, 1974.

Rothbaum, D., *et al.*: Echocardiographic manifestations of right sinus of Valsalva aneurysm. Circulation, *49*:768, 1974.

Shaub, M., Wilson, R., and Young, G.: Echocardiographic diagnosis of supravalvular aortic stenosis: A case report. J. Clin. Ultrasound, *3*:2, 1975.

Spangler, R., *et al.*: Echocardiographic demonstration of bacterial vegetations in active infective endocarditis. J. Clin. Ultrasound, *1*:126, 1973.

Usher, B., Goulden, D., and Murgo, J. P.: Echocardiographic detection of supravalvular aortic stenosis. Circulation, *49*:1257, 1974.

Vredevoe, L., Creekmore, S., and Schiller, N.: The measurement of systolic time intervals by echocardiography. J. Clin. Ultrasound, *2*:99, 1974.

Wray, T.: Echocardiographic manifestations of flail aortic valve leaflets in bacterial endocarditis. Circulation, *51*:832, 1975.

Yuste, P., *et al.*: Dissecting aortic aneurysm diagnosed by echocardiography. Br. Heart J., *36*:111, 1974.

5

TRICUSPID VALVE

Normal Tricuspid Valve

The usual method of locating an anterior tricuspid leaflet is first to find the aortic root. Then the transducer should be turned directly medially into the sternum and tilted slightly inferiorly toward the patient's right foot. If the characteristic motion similar to that of a normal mitral valve is not seen, the maneuver should be repeated, the angle being modified somewhat. A point of confusion occasionally arises as to whether the tricuspid or the pulmonary valve motion is

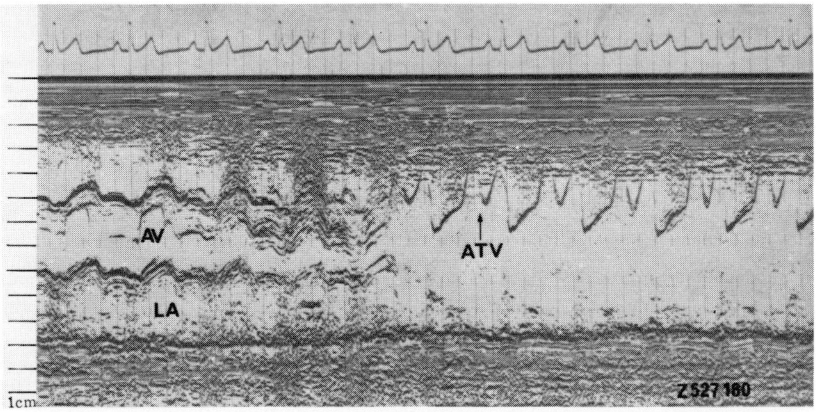

Figure 61. Scan from aorta to tricuspid valve. Tricuspid valve appears to be much closer to the transducer. This is one way to differentiate tricuspid from mitral valve; the latter lies deeper in the chest and therefore is farther from transducer. AV = aortic valve, LA = left atrium and ATV = anterior tricuspid valve.

being recorded. Under certain circumstances the motion may appear to be similar. The examiner should check the direction in which the transducer is pointing to confirm which valve is being recorded. One must point medially to locate the tricuspid valve. The pulmonary valve is never found in this position in a heart with normal anatomical relationships (Figure 61).

To make a more extensive check of the anatomical relationships of the tricuspid to the mitral valve, the transducer may be angled from a medial to a lateral position. In so doing, the ultrasound beam passes from the tricuspid valve across the septum and laterally into the mitral valve. Figure 62 shows this relationship of the tricuspid and mitral valves to the transducer.

Adequate tricuspid valves may be recorded either through the sternum or in children from the right sternal border. If the heart is positioned very low in the chest, subxiphoid approaches to the tricuspid valve are also useful (see Figure 119*C*).

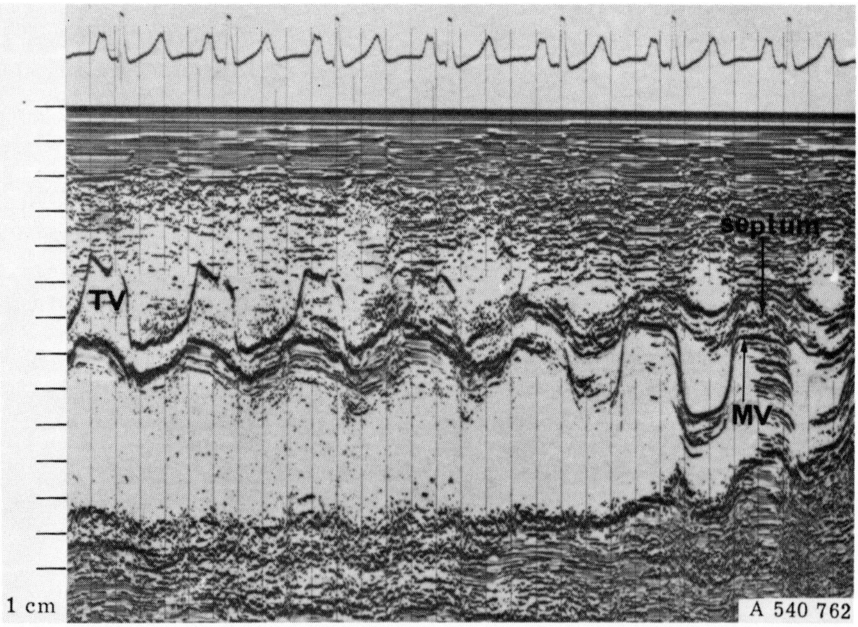

Figure 62. Scan from tricuspid valve across interventricular septum to mitral valve. Transducer was angled from medial to lateral position along left sternal border. Cardiac catheterization revealed severe mitral stenosis, with both mild mitral and tricuspid insufficiency. Cardiac output was estimated at 2.9 L/min with an index of 1.6 L/min/M². TV = tricuspid valve and MV = mitral valve.

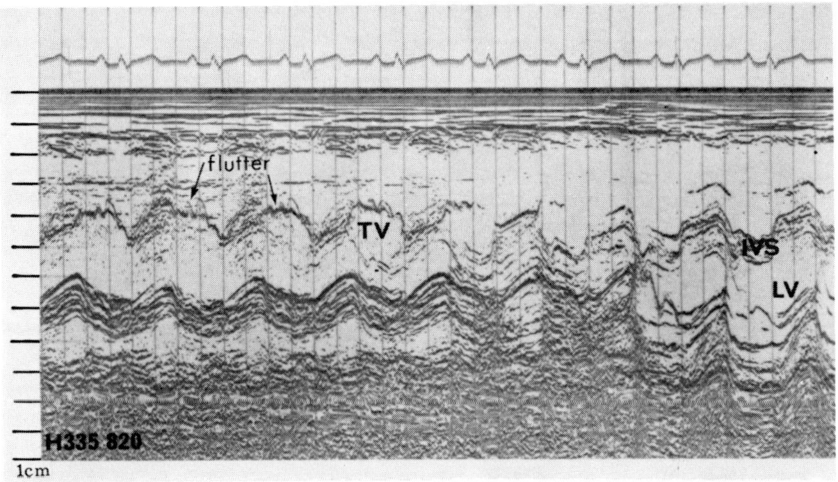

Figure 63. Patient, age 24, with history of two faulty fascia lata repairs for congenital pulmonary stenosis. Pulmonary valve was finally excised, leaving massive pulmonary insufficiency. TV = tricuspid valve, IVS = interventricular septum, and LV=left ventricle.

Fluttering: Pulmonary Insufficiency

The tricuspid valve will respond to pulmonary insufficiency in the same way that the mitral valve responds to aortic insufficiency, *i.e.*, the valve flutters, and the diastolic closing slope is reduced (Figure 63). The normal motion of the anterior tricuspid leaflet is altered because of the normal flow of blood from the right atrium mixing with the regurgitant jet of pulmonary insufficiency, creating marked turbulence. The tricuspid valve itself is not diseased but merely reflects a pattern of motion produced by another valvular lesion. Other investigators report that tricuspid valve fluttering does not always occur in pulmonary insufficiency. This has also been noted in our laboratory.

Elevated Right Ventricular End-diastolic Pressure

Right ventricular end-diastolic pressure may be evaluated from the motion of the tricuspid valve in the same way that left ventricular end-diastolic pressure is evaluated from the mitral valve. Both anterior and posterior leaflets of the tricuspid valve must be recorded from atrial contraction to actual closure. The leaflets must be seen to *meet* at the C point (Figure 64).

The A-C interval is subtracted from the P-R interval on the electrocardiogram, and the P-R interval remaining should be greater than 0.06 sec for the right ventricular end-diastolic pressure to be regarded as normal. These intervals are easier to measure if the paper speed is at least 50 mm/sec, and time lines are set at 0.1 sec. Individuals

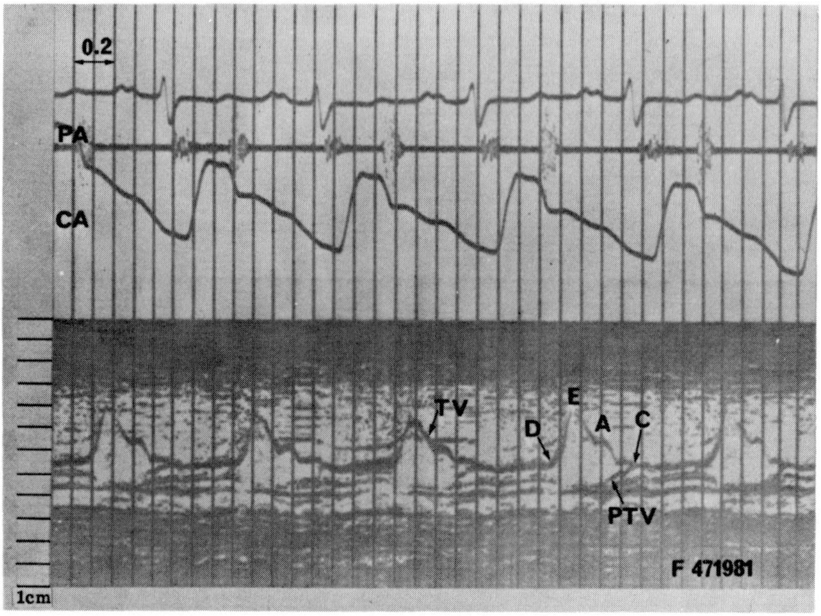

Figure 64. Tricuspid valve from patient with renal disease and cardiomyopathy. No catheterization was performed. PA=phonocardiogram from pulmonary artery, CA=carotid pulse tracing, TV=tricuspid valve, D= initial point of opening of tricuspid valve, E=maximum point of opening amplitude, A=peak of atrial contraction and C=closure of valve.

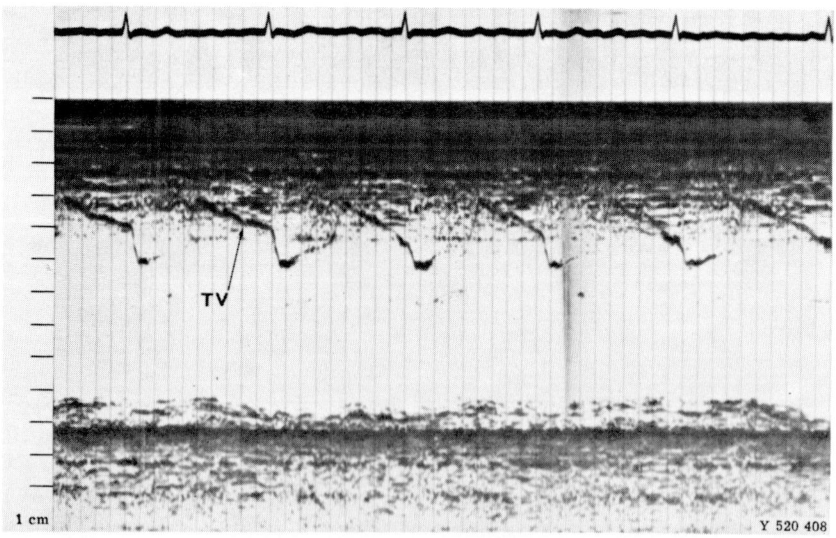

Figure 65. Patient, age 53, with documented moderate, noncalcific mitral stenosis, minimal to mild aortic insufficiency and minimal tricuspid insufficiency with mild pulmonary hypertension. There was no gradient across tricuspid valve. Cardiac output was calculated to be 3.2 L/min with an index of 2.1 L/min/M^2. TV = tricuspid valve.

with long P-R intervals will have mitral and tricuspid valves that appear to have long closure times, but by completion of the standard measurements, the remaining P-R interval should indicate the approximate right or left ventricular end-diastolic pressure. An important rule to keep in mind is *not* to draw a conclusion on valve motion from guesswork; make the measurement before passing judgment.

Tricuspid Stenosis

A very difficult diagnosis to make is the evaluation of tricuspid stenosis. Because the pressures in the right heart are low, it is possible for the valve to be badly diseased and yet produce no pressure gradient at cardiac catheterization.

Figure 65 was taken from a patient brought to catheterization for evaluation of mitral stenosis. The tricuspid valve pattern of motion does not appear thickened either in this echogram or in subsequent tracings taken a few days later. The closing velocity of the valve does appear reduced. There was no gradient measured across this valve at catheterization.

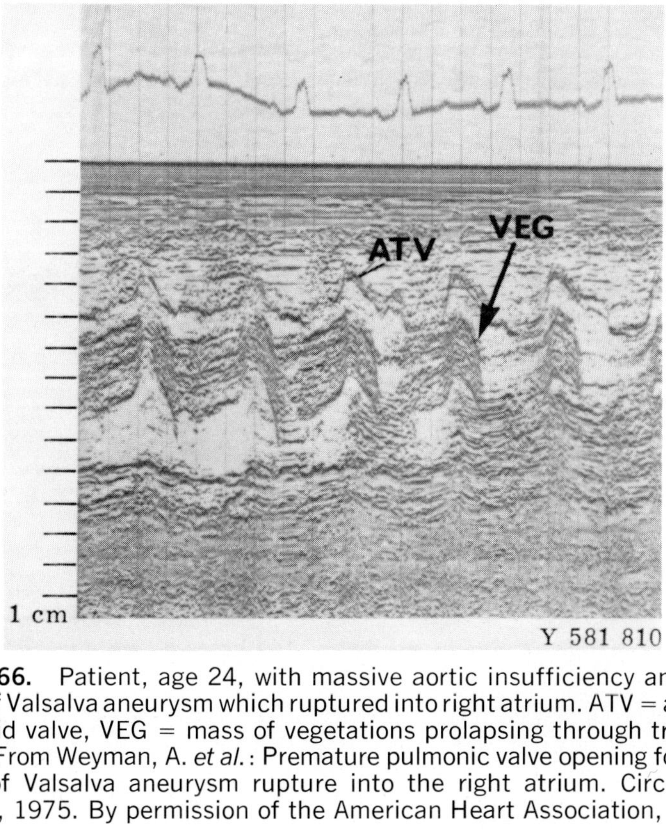

Figure 66. Patient, age 24, with massive aortic insufficiency and large sinus of Valsalva aneurysm which ruptured into right atrium. ATV = anterior tricuspid valve, VEG = mass of vegetations prolapsing through tricuspid valve. (From Weyman, A. *et al.*: Premature pulmonic valve opening following sinus of Valsalva aneurysm rupture into the right atrium. Circulation, *51*:556, 1975. By permission of the American Heart Association, Inc.)

The tricuspid valve echograms of other patients have been similar to Figure 65, and pressure gradients have been recorded. The examiner cannot reliably predict when a pressure gradient will be present from the motion of the tricuspid valve.

Ruptured Sinus of Valsalva Aneurysm

Figure 66 is from a patient with catheterization and surgically proven ruptured sinus of Valsalva aneurysm into the right atrium secondary to subacute bacterial endocarditis. The arrow indicates a large mass moving within the tricuspid orifice. This was a large vegetative mass attached to the aortic leaflet, and it was prolapsing from the right atrium through the tricuspid valve. The standard technique was used to record the tricuspid valve motion (see p. 67).

Some right atrial tumors prolapsing from the right atrium through the tricuspid valve into the right ventricle may produce a tracing resembling Figure 66.

Suggested Reading

Chandraratna, P., *et al.*: Echocardiographic detection of tricuspid valve prolapse. Circulation, *51*:823, 1975.

Green, E., Agruss, N., and Adolph, R.: Right-sided Austin-Flint murmur: Documentation of intracardiac phonocardiography, echocardiography and postmortem findings. Am. J. Cardiol., *32*:370, 1973.

Joyner, C., *et al.*: Reflected ultrasound in the diagnosis of tricuspid stenosis. Am. J. Cardiol., *19*:66, 1967.

Kotler, M., and Lundstrom, N.: Tricuspid valve in Ebstein's anomaly. Circulation, *49*:194, 1974 (letter).

Lee, C., *et al.*: Detection of tricuspid valve vegetations by echocardiography. Chest, *66*:432, 1974.

Lundstrom, N.: Echocardiography in the diagnosis of Ebstein's anomaly of the tricuspid valve. Circulation, *47*:597, 1973.

Nanda, N., Gramiak, R., and Manning, J.: Echocardiography of the tricuspid valve in congenital left ventricular-right atrial communication. Circulation, *51*:268, 1975.

Nanda, N., *et al.*: Echocardiographic features of subpulmonic obstruction in dextro-transposition of the great vessels. Circulation, *51*:515, 1975.

Nimura, Y., *et al.*: The ultrasound cardiogram of the tricuspid valve in healthy subjects. Jap. Heart J., *13*:394, 1972.

Tavel, M., *et al.*: Opening snap of the tricuspid valve in atrial septal defect: A phonocardiographic and reflected ultrasound study of sounds in relationship to movements of the tricuspid valve. Am. Heart J., *80*:555, 1970.

6

PULMONARY VALVE

The posterior leaflet of the pulmonary valve lies superior to the mitral valve, or lateral and superior in relation to the aortic valve. Usually the pulmonary valve motion may be recorded by gradual tilting of the transducer superiorly from the mitral valve. If it cannot be recorded by this technique, then the transducer should be repositioned one intercostal space higher, close to the sternum to avoid the lung. The patient should be supine rather than in a left lateral position (Figure 67).

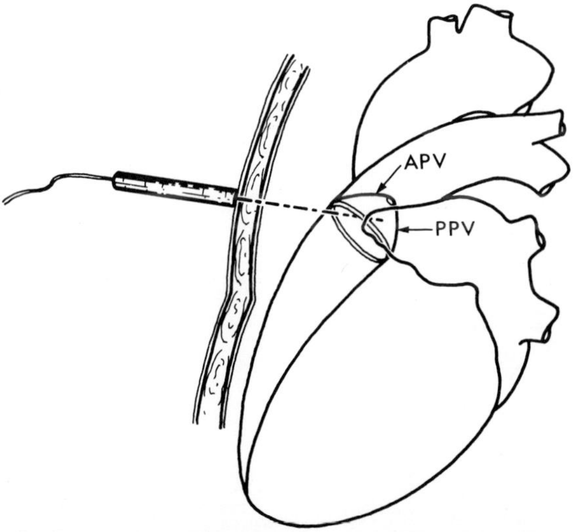

Figure 67. Position of transducer in relation to pulmonary valve. APV=anterior pulmonary valve and PPV=posterior pulmonary valve. (From Weyman, A., *et al.*: Echocardiographic patterns of pulmonary valve motion in valvular pulmonary stenosis. Am. J. Cardiol., *34*:644, 1974.)

Once the pulmonary leaflet has been recorded, its relationship to the aortic valve may be established by tipping the transducer slightly inferiorly and medially toward the right shoulder. Figure 68 demonstrates the results of this technique. The dotted line shows the posterior pulmonary leaflet to lie in a plane with the anterior aortic wall. The aortic valve lies more deeply in the chest and is confined by the anterior and posterior aortic walls. There is a definite mass of tissue posterior to the pulmonary valve which is not present posterior to the aorta.

The mass of tissue behind the pulmonary valve should not be mistaken for tumor material, which may be present in patients with left atrial myxomas. These tumors may be verified by tilting the transducer from the area of the aortic valve inferiorly into the mitral valve (Figures 69 and 70).

Figures 69 and 70 were taken from a patient with a proven left atrial myxoma. In Figure 69 the transducer is angled high into the aortic area; the myxoma is seen as a dense mass behind the posterior wall of the aorta.

In Figure 70 the transducer is tilted inferiorly and laterally into the mitral valve. The tumor is seen to persist in the mitral orifice during diastole. One can see that the mitral valve opens rapidly, and a short time later the tumor prolapses into the orifice, thus obstructing blood flow and causing the mitral valve motion to mimic mitral stenosis.

At no time has the transducer been angled superiorly in the direction of the pulmonary valve. The dense echoes in Figures 69 and 70 are from tumor material, not the naturally occurring tissue that lies posterior to the pulmonary valve.

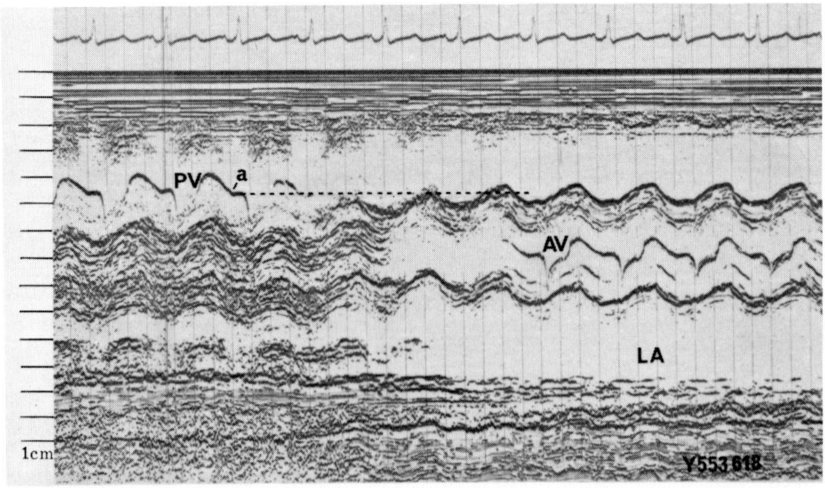

Figure 68. Scan from pulmonary to aortic valve. PV = pulmonary valve, a = atrial contraction response, AV = aortic valve and LA = left atrium.

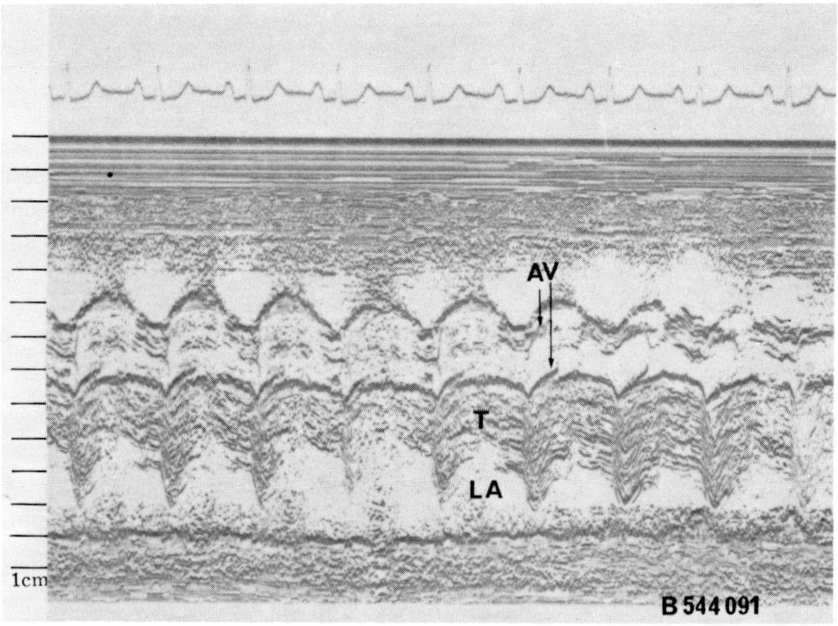

Figure 69. Left atrial myxoma seen up against posterior aortic wall. AV = aortic valve, T = tumor and LA = left atrium.

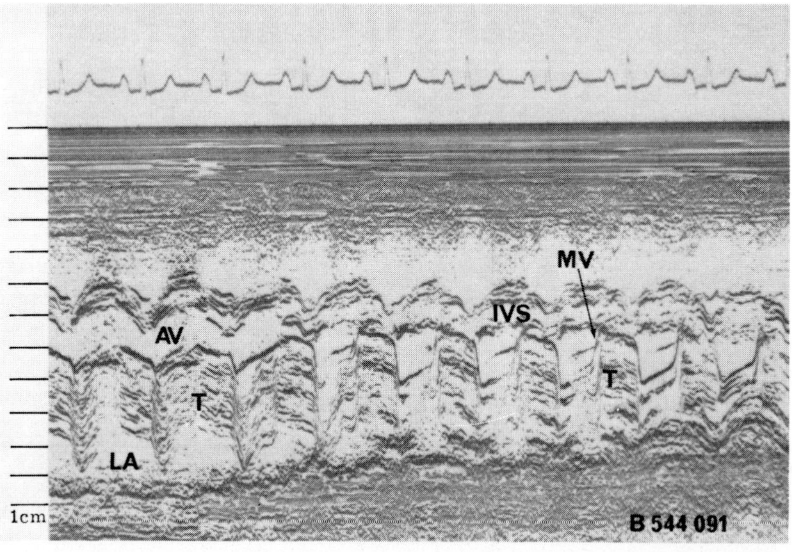

Figure 70. Scan from aorta and left atrium inferior to mitral valve. AV = aortic valve, LA = left atrium, T = tumor, IVS = interventricular septum and MV = mitral valve.

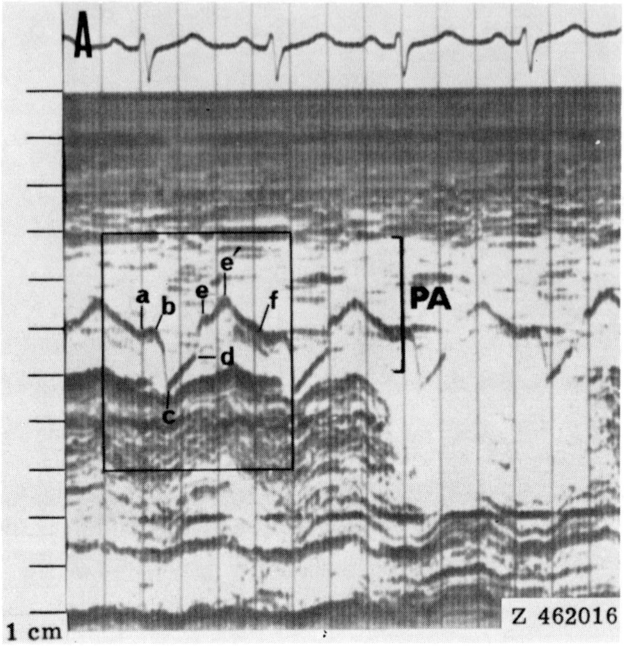

Figure 71. Normal motion of pulmonary valve throughout diastole and systole. e–f = diastole, a = atrial contraction, b–c = onset of systole, blood flows into main pulmonary artery, c–d = mid-to-late systole and PA = pulmonary artery. (From Weyman, A., *et al.*: Echocardiographic patterns of pulmonary valve motion in valvular pulmonary stenosis. Am. J. Cardiol., *34*:644, 1974.)

Normal Pulmonary Valve

In the adult patient the posterior leaflet of the pulmonary valve is the only one perpendicular to the sound beam. The anterior leaflet is parallel to the sound beam and cannot be recorded except rarely. The posterior leaflet appears thin and pliable even when diseased.

That part of the leaflet most often recorded from healthy subjects is reflected in Figure 71. The depth of the *a* wave may range from 3 to 7 mm in valves that are normal or mildly stenotic.

The novice may mistakenly identify the tricuspid as the pulmonary valve. When one is considering what valve is being recorded, the examiner should identify the position toward which the transducer is pointed. If the transducer is angled medially toward the sternum, the tricuspid valve is being recorded. If the transducer is pointed in a plane with the left eye, the pulmonary valve is being recorded. The examiner should always know what angle he was pointing when valvular structures were being recorded.

The difference between tricuspid and pulmonary valves may be established at the time the tracing is being interpreted. If the valve is tricuspid, the *a* wave should move anteriorly toward the transducer shortly after the P wave on the electrocardiogram (Figure 72).

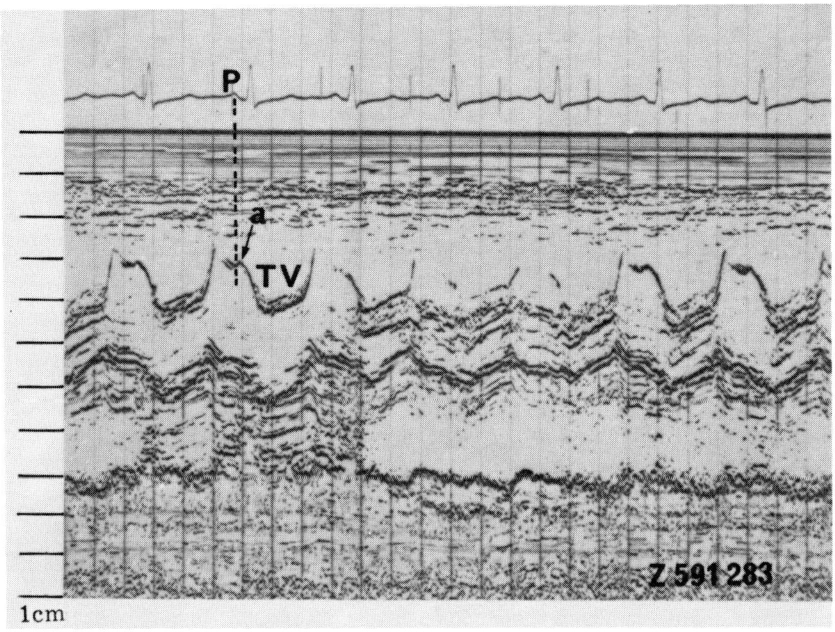

Figure 72. Normal tricuspid valve from patient with prolapsing mitral valve. Transducer is directed medially toward sternum. a=response to atrial contraction, P=P wave and TV=tricuspid valve.

If the valve is pulmonary, the *a* wave should move away from the transducer near the end of the P wave on the electrocardiogram. At no time has the *a* wave of the pulmonary valve been observed to move anteriorly toward the transducer shortly after the onset of the P wave on the electrocardiogram. It may move toward the transducer, however, just prior to the onset of systole, timed at the end of the QRS wave on the electrocardiogram.

Pulmonary Stenosis

Moderate pulmonary stenosis may drive the *a* wave to a depth of 13 mm with partial return of the valve toward the baseline before the onset of systole.

Severe pulmonary stenosis will cause the pulmonary valve to open completely with the onset of systole; the *a* wave will appear to be absent because it never returns toward the baseline before the onset of systole. In fact the valve appears to be fully open before systole occurs. Hypertrophy of the right ventricular wall and dilatation of the right ventricular dimension may occur in severe pulmonary stenosis, although exceptions have been noted.

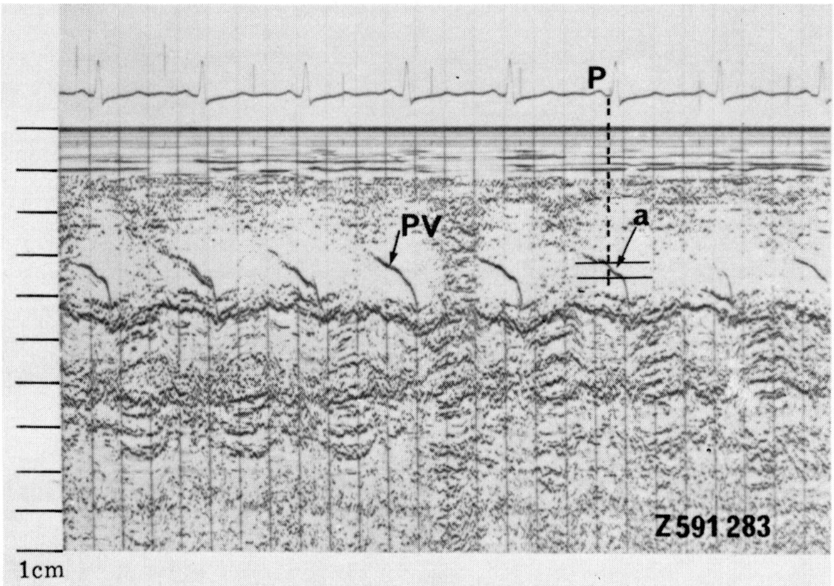

Figure 73. Normal pulmonary valve from same patient as in Figure 72. The late diastolic and early systolic motion of valve is most common portion of valve which can be recorded. PV = pulmonary valve, a = response to atrial contraction and P = P wave.

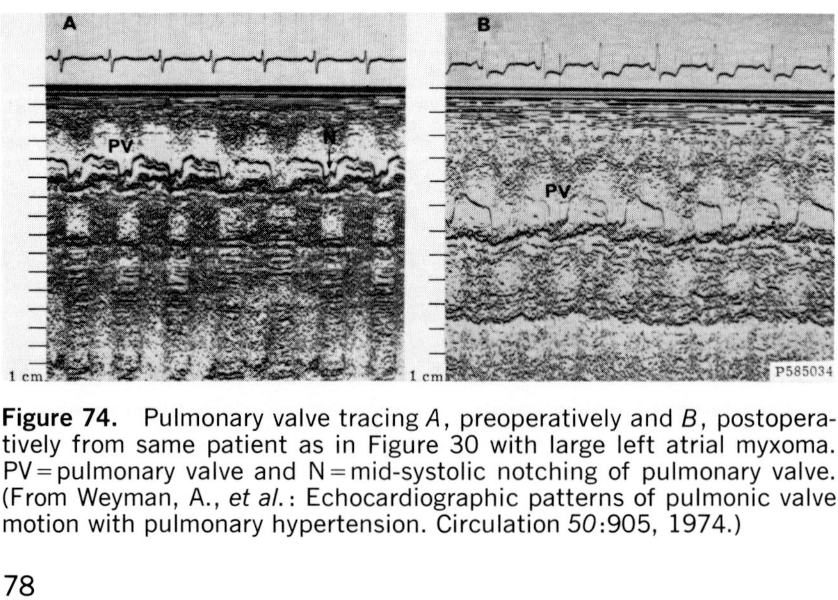

Figure 74. Pulmonary valve tracing *A*, preoperatively and *B*, postoperatively from same patient as in Figure 30 with large left atrial myxoma. PV = pulmonary valve and N = mid-systolic notching of pulmonary valve. (From Weyman, A., *et al.*: Echocardiographic patterns of pulmonic valve motion with pulmonary hypertension. Circulation *50*:905, 1974.)

Pulmonary Hypertension and Atrial Fibrillation

With the presence of significant pulmonary hypertension, the *a* wave excursion will be reduced from 0 to 2 mm. The e′–f slope may be flattened, and there usually is a notching effect (N) in the systolic c–d slope (Figure 74). These findings are reported in the literature.

Figure 74 is a tracing from a woman with a very large left atrial myxoma. Figure 74*A*, of the pulmonary valve, indicates that significant pulmonary hypertension is present as seen in the absence of *a* waves and mid-systolic notching. Several weeks following removal of the tumor, the pulmonary valve tracing in Figure 74*B* shows the e′–f slope to be increased and absence of the mid-systolic notch, indicating a drop in pulmonary pressures. Pulmonary pressures were not obtained; the patient refused preoperative cardiac catheterization.

In atrial fibrillation, since there is no P wave on the electrocardiogram, there will be no *a* wave response seen on the pulmonary valve.

Suggested Reading

Chung, K., *et al.*: Echocardiography in truncus arteriosus: The value of pulmonic valve detection. Circulation, *48*:281, 1973.

Goodman, D., Harrison, D., and Popp, R.: Echocardiographic features of primary pulmonary hypertension. Am. J. Cardiol., *33*:438, 1974.

Gramiak, R., Nanda, N., and Shah, P.: Echocardiographic detection of pulmonary valve. Radiology, *102*:153, 1972.

Nanda, N., *et al.*: Evaluation of pulmonary hypertension by echocardiography. J. Clin. Ultrasound, *1*:255, 1973.

Nanda, N., *et al.*: Echocardiographic evaluation of pulmonary hypertension. Circulation, *50*:575, 1974.

Nanda, N., *et al.*: Echocardiographic diagnosis of pulmonary hypertension. Excerpta Medica., *277*:12, 1973.

Sakamoto, T., *et al.*: Echocardiogram of the pulmonic valve. Jap. Heart J., *15*:360, 1974.

Weyman, A., *et al.*: Echocardiographic patterns of pulmonic valve motion in pulmonic stenosis. Am. J. Cardiol., *34*:644, 1974.

Weyman, A., *et al.*: Echocardiographic patterns of pulmonary valve motion with pulmonary hypertension. Circulation, *50*:905, 1974.

Weyman, A., *et al.*: Premature pulmonic valve opening following sinus of Valsalva aneurysm rupture into the right atrium. Circulation, *51*:556, 1975.

Weyman, A., *et al.*: Echocardiographic differentiation of infundibular from valvular pulmonic stenosis. Am. J. Cardiol., *36*:98, 1975.

7

PROSTHETIC AORTIC AND MITRAL BALL VALVES

Examination of prosthetic valves is intriguing. The two valves with which this laboratory has had the most experience are the mitral and aortic Starr-Edwards ball valves. Other types of valves such as the Beall, Bjork-Shiley, Lillehei-Kaster, Cutter-Smeloff, fascia lata homografts and, most recently, Hancock valves have come through in very small numbers, and they were recorded but not described concerning functional status.

Single examinations do not contribute much information on the function of the valve motion. Serial studies should be the rule, the first study being initiated 5 to 7 days postoperatively and thereafter as often as the patient returns to outpatient clinics. Whereas a single echogram of a prosthetic valve may give little information regarding the functional status, serial examinations may reflect remarkable changes.

To examine the aortic Starr-Edwards prosthesis, the transducer should be positioned in the supraclavicular position (Figure 75) or in the second intercostal space along the right sternal border. The ultrasound beam should be perpendicular to the ball as it opens, moving toward the transducer during systole (Figure 76*A*, arrow). The ball remains open as long as an adequate volume of blood passes into the aorta, then moves to a closed position at the end of systole. If the ball motion cannot be obtained from this position, then the transducer should be placed at the apex and angled through the long axis of the left ventricle. The motion of the ball will be exactly opposite to that seen

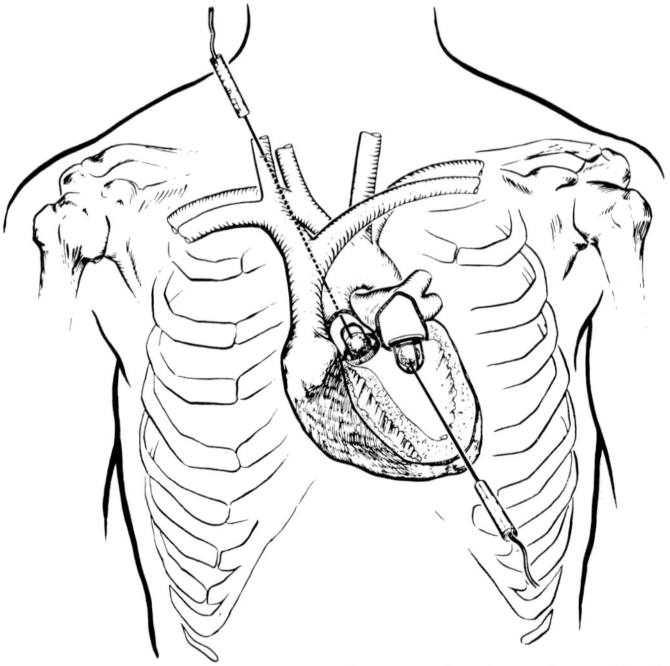

Figure 75. Placement of transducer for examination of prosthetic mitral and aortic valves. (From Schuchman, H., *et al.*: Intracavitary echoes in patients with mitral prosthetic valves. J. Clin. Ultrasound, *3*:107, 1975, No. 2.)

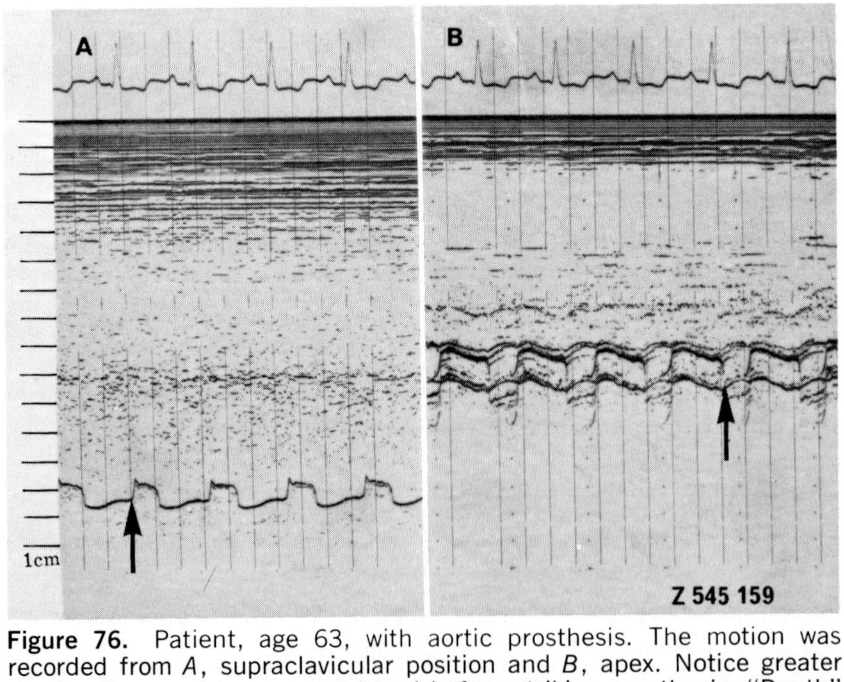

Figure 76. Patient, age 63, with aortic prosthesis. The motion was recorded from *A*, supraclavicular position and *B*, apex. Notice greater depth ultrasound beam must travel before striking prosthesis. "Depth" must be compressed when one examines prosthetic aortic valves from supraclavicular position; otherwise they will neither be seen on oscilloscope nor recorded on paper.

from the supraclavicular position, *i.e.*, the ball will move away from the transducer with the onset of systole (Figure 76*B*, arrow) and return toward the transducer at the completion of systole.

The effects of serial examinations may be seen in Figure 77 as the function of the valve becomes altered. Figure 77*A* was taken from a patient several days postoperatively. The aortic ball motion was recorded from the apex. The ball moves to an open position (arrow), stays open without any oscillation during systole and then closes, moving toward the transducer.

Four months later, Figure 77*B* was recorded. A murmur, indicating aortic insufficiency, was heard. The ball motion was again recorded from the apical position. One can now see many oscillations during systole (arrow). The patient was not catheterized to establish the degree of aortic insufficiency. It is significant that the change is recorded so readily from one interval when the valve function appeared to be normal to a later date when dysfunction began.

The mitral Starr-Edwards prosthesis is examined by placing the transducer at the apex (Figure 78) and directing the sound beam

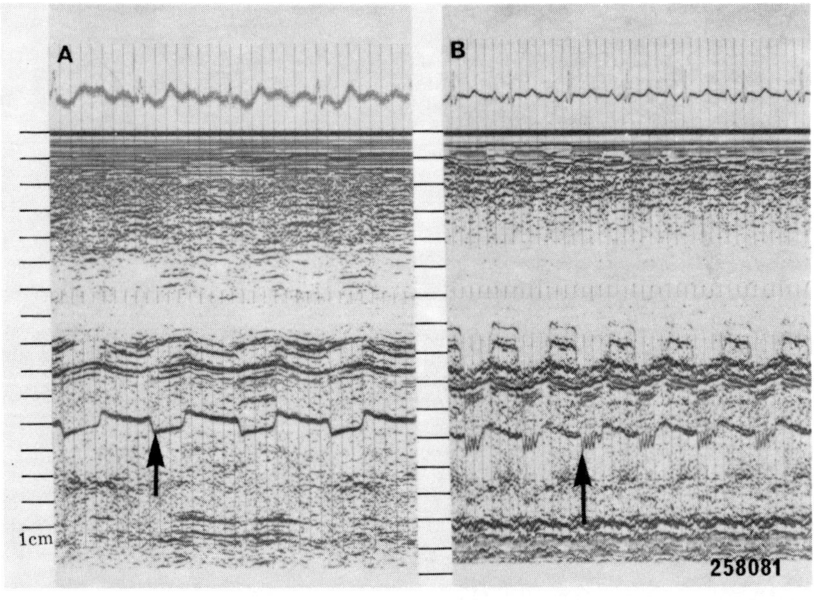

Figure 77. Patient, age 50, with aortic Starr-Edwards prosthesis. Tracing *B* was recorded four months after tracing *A*, demonstrating change in valvular function of unclear cause. Prosthesis may be responding to newly heard murmur of aortic insufficiency, or flutter during systole may be attributable to low cardiac output. Volume of blood may not be enough to support prosthetic ball in open position throughout systole. Patient had associated residual moderate mitral stenosis following mitral commissurotomy at time of aortic valve replacement.

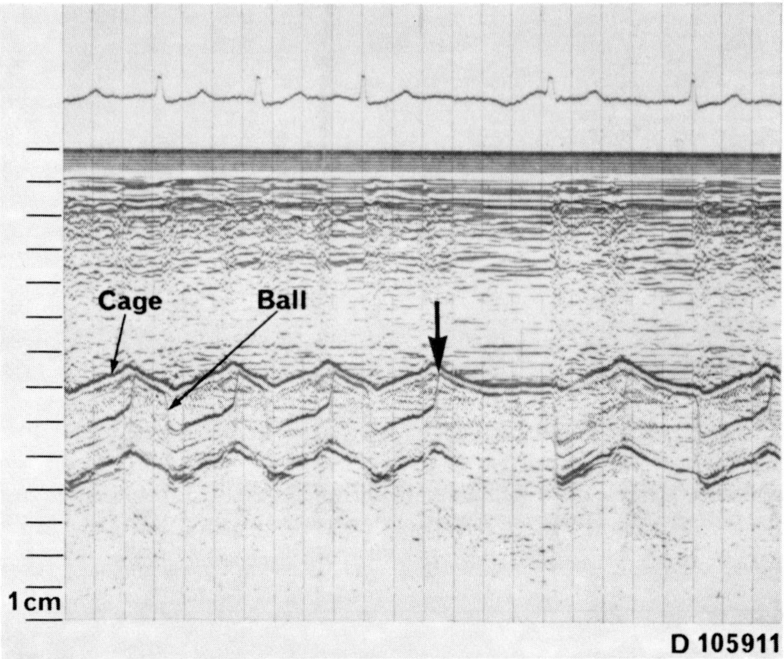

Figure 78. Mitral valve prosthesis, replaced in 1972; 38-year-old patient has remained without symptoms since operation. Left atrial dimension is dilated at 6.0 cm. (From Schuchman, H., *et al.*: Intracavitary echoes in patients with mitral prosthetic valves. J. Clin. Ultrasound, *3*:107, 1975, No. 2.)

perpendicularly to the movement of the ball as it opens during diastole (heavy arrow), remaining open throughout diastole and then closing prior to systole. The *reject* of the echographic instrument is set at very low levels (position 1) so that any low intensity matter which may be floating within the left ventricular cavity may be recorded.

A normally functioning mitral prosthesis is shown in Figure 78. The echoes representing the cage and ball are well defined by reducing the coarse gain.

A significant number of patients have exhibited extraneous echoes moving at very high velocities anterior to the mitral prosthesis. The transducer was positioned at the apex and the reject set on position 1 to detect these very low intensity echoes. These echoes (Figure 79, arrowheads) were noted to move from the mitral valve toward the apex, then away from the transducer toward the left ventricular outflow tract.

A study was undertaken to examine this phenomenon concerning the origin of these particles. It was noted that these echoes occurred in patients seen shortly postoperatively when fibrinous infiltration of the prosthesis was taking place. These echoes may have been caused by

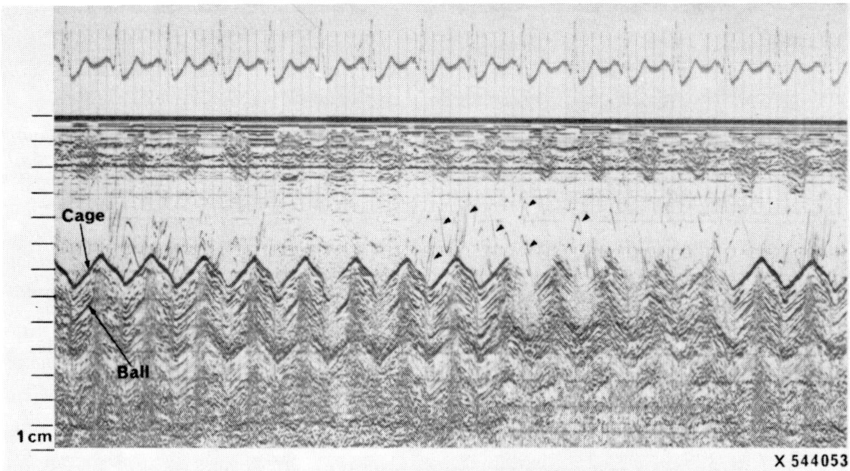

Figure 79. Second of three mitral prostheses placed in 20-year-old patient between February and September, 1973. All three valves showed high-velocity echoes anterior to prosthesis. Patient died 6 months after placement of third prosthesis. (From Schuchman, H., *et al.*: Intracavitary echoes in patients with mitral prosthetic valves. J. Clin. Ultrasound, *3*:107, 1975, No. 2.)

some of this material breaking away from the prosthesis. These echoes were also visualized in several patients who underwent surgical treatment for deterioration of cloth-covered mitral prostheses. We could not definitely pinpoint the origin of these echoes, although the study raised some interesting ideas which deserve followup. The most significant finding was the presence of symptoms in patients who exhibited this peculiar phenomenon.

The patient whose tracing is seen in Figure 79 sustained the replacement of three mitral prostheses and one aortic prosthesis. Two of the mitral prostheses were replaced because of massive mitral insufficiency. Notations were made of the appearance of the mitral prostheses at the time of reoperation. About the first prosthesis the surgeon's report stated in part: ". . . the cause of the mitral valve insufficiency was extensive clotting and not due to any perivalvular leak." About the second prosthesis: "The valve was partially dehisced from the annulus . . . extending over a distance of about 3 cm. In addition, there was a great deal of clot on the valve."

Echocardiographic examination of this patient 3 months following implantation of the third prosthesis again disclosed high velocity echoes anterior to the mitral prosthesis. However, fluoroscopic examination indicated normal excursions of the mitral valve, and the patient demonstrated no further cardiac deterioration. The patient died 6 months later, of liver failure. Autopsy was not performed.

Suggested Reading

Alderman, E., *et al.*: Normal and prosthetic atrioventricular valve motion in atrial flutter. Circulation, *45*:1206, 1972.

Assad-Morell, J., *et al.*: Malfunctioning tricuspid valve prosthesis. Clinical, phonocardiographic, echocardiographic and surgical findings. Mayo Clin. Proc., *42*:443, 1974.

Belenkie, I., *et al.*: Malfunction of a Cutter-Smeloff mitral ball valve prosthesis: Diagnosis by phonocardiography and echocardiography. Am. Heart J., *86*:339, 1973.

Ben-Zvi, J., *et al.*: Thrombosis on Bjork-Shiley aortic valve prosthesis: Clinical, arteriographic, echocardiographic and therapeutic observations in seven cases. Am. J. Cardiol., *34*:538, 1974.

Douglas, J., and Williams, G.: Echocardiographic evaluation of the Bjork-Shiley prosthetic valve. Circulation, *50*:52, 1974.

Gibson, T., *et al.*: Echocardiographic and phonocardiographic characteristics of the Lillehei-Kaster mitral valve prosthesis. Circulation, *49*:434, 1974.

Gimenez, J., *et al.*: Dynamics of the Starr-Edwards ball valve prosthesis: A cinefluorographic and ultrasonic study in humans. Am. J. Med. Sci., *250*:652, 1965.

Horowitz, M., Goodman, D., and Popp, R.: Echocardiographic diagnosis of calcific stenosis of a stented aortic homograft in the mitral position. J. Clin. Ultrasound, *2*:179, 1974.

Illmurzynska, K., and Kompiel, J.: Ultrasonographic studies of implanted valves. Kardiol. Pol., *15*:445, 1972.

Johnson, M., Holmes, J., and Paton, B.: Echocardiographic determination of mitral disc valve excursion. Circulation, *47*:1274, 1973.

Johnson, M., Paton, B., and Holmes, J.: Ultrasonic evaluation of prosthetic valve motion. Circulation, *41*(II):3, 1970.

Mahringer, W., and Hausen, W.: Ultrasound cardiogram in patients with mitral valve disc prostheses. Angiology, *21*:336, 1970.

Mary, D., *et al.*: Echocardiographic studies of stented fascia lata grafts in the mitral position. Circulation, *49*:237, 1974.

Miller, H., Gibson, D., and Stephens, J.: Role of echocardiography and phonocardiography in the diagnosis of mitral paraprosthetic regurgitation with Starr-Edwards prostheses. Br. Heart J., *35*:1217, 1973.

Miller, H., Stephens, J., and Gibson, D.: Echocardiographic features of mitral Starr-Edwards paraprosthetic regurgitation. Br. Heart J., *35*:560, 1973.

Nanda, N., *et al.*: Echocardiographic assessment of left ventricular outflow width in the selection of mitral valve prosthesis. Circulation, *48*:1208, 1973.

Oliva, P., *et al.*: Dysfunction of the Beall mitral prosthesis and its detection by cinefluoroscopy and echocardiography. Am. J. Cardiol., *31*:393, 1973.

Pfeifer, J., *et al.*: Malfunction of mitral ball valve prosthesis due to thrombus. Am. J. Cardiol., *29*:95, 1972.

Popp, R., and Carmichael, B.: Cardiac echography in the diagnosis of prosthetic mitral valve malfunction. Circulation, *44*(II):33, 1971.

Schelbert, H., and Muller, O.: Detection of fungal vegetations involving a Starr-Edwards mitral prosthesis by means of ultrasound. Vasc. Surg., *6*:20, 1972.

Schuchman, H., *et al.*: Intracavitary echoes in patients with mitral prosthetic valves. J. Clin. Ultrasound, *3*:2, 1975.

Sgarbi, E., *et al.*: Ultrasonocardiographic evaluation of functional capacity in persons with valve prosthesis. Boll. Soc. Ital. Cardiol., *16*:675, 1971.

Siggers, D., and Srivongse, S.: Analysis of dynamics of mitral Starr-Edwards valve prosthesis using reflected ultrasound. Br. Heart J., *32*:552, 1970.

Siggers, D., Srivongse, S., and Deuchar, D.: Analysis of dynamics of mitral Starr-Edwards valve prosthesis using reflected ultrasound. Br. Heart J., *33*:401, 1971.

Suwansirikul, S., *et al.*: Late thrombosis of Starr-Edwards tricuspid ball valve prothesis. Am. J. Cardiol., *34*:737, 1974.

Watts, E., Abdel-Mohsen, N., and Barnes, R.: Echocardiography in evaluation of mitral valve prostheses. J. Clin. Ultrasound, *3*:2, 1975.

Yuste, P., *et al.*: Mitral prosthesis and left ventricular function. Ultrasonic study. Rev. Esp. Cardiol., *27*:157, 1974.

8

LEFT VENTRICLE

Left Ventricular Study

A satisfactory left ventricular study is one that can be reproduced on multiple occasions and by different examiners. To do this, specific structures of the left ventricle must be recorded simultaneously. The technique to record these structures is the same regardless of the type of disease or the status of the left ventricular function.

Every adequate left ventricular study must have the right and left sides of the septum, some portion of both mitral cusps and endocardial and pericardial surfaces of the free posterior left ventricular wall. The examiner is so limited as to where all of these structures may be simultaneously recorded that the plane from which one records is almost identical in serial studies.

Figure 80 is an accurate left ventricular study from a subject without heart disease. The right ventricular dimension measures 1.4 cm. Should the right ventricle become dilated, the dimension may then measure 2.6 to 3.0 cm or greater; the direction of the septal motion may change as well.

The left ventricular dimension measures 5.0 cm. Should the left ventricle dilate, the measurement would be greater than the acceptable normal limits. The left ventricular wall motion may be altered by abnormalities such as coronary artery disease, left ventricular volume overloads, myopathy, arrhythmia, pericardial effusion or operation. If dimensions are borderline between normal and abnormal, they should be divided by the body surface area of the patient.

Most left ventricular studies are improved if the patient is positioned slightly left laterally. After mitral valve tracing has been obtained,

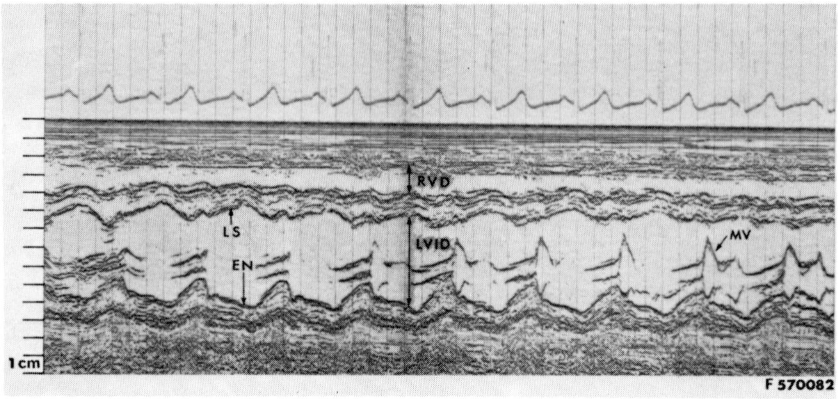

Figure 80. Normal scan from deep in left ventricle to mitral valve. RVD = right ventricular dimension, LVID = left ventricular internal dimension, LS = left septum, EN = endocardial surface of posterior left ventricular wall and MV=mitral valve.

the transducer should be angled slightly inferiorly and laterally from the valve to obtain the best tracing of the posterior left ventricular wall and left septum. The septum and posterior wall will then become well defined. At this point some repositioning of the transducer may be needed. If the septum is persistently broken up—regardless of how inferiorly and laterally the examiner is pointing the probe—the transducer should be moved either closer to the sternum or toward a higher or lower intercostal space, or both. Most examiners with whom I have worked tend to place the transducer too laterally and too low on the chest.

Positional Change of Transducer

In Figure 81*A* the transducer was placed in the third intercostal space. Inspiration caused the lung to move between the transducer and the heart.

To correct this problem the transducer was moved to the fourth intercostal space. Correction of respiratory interference may be achieved on other patients by sliding the transducer nearer to the sternum or by turning the patient slightly left laterally, thus rolling the lung laterally. If nothing else works, have the patient expel his air and hold his breath to achieve a tracing that is free of respiratory interference (Figure 81*B*).

Positional Change of Patient

Initially most echocardiographic examinations are begun with the patient supine. Not infrequently the resulting tracing of the left ventricle resembles Figure 82*A*. The septum is poorly defined, and in addition, the coarse gain setting is too high.

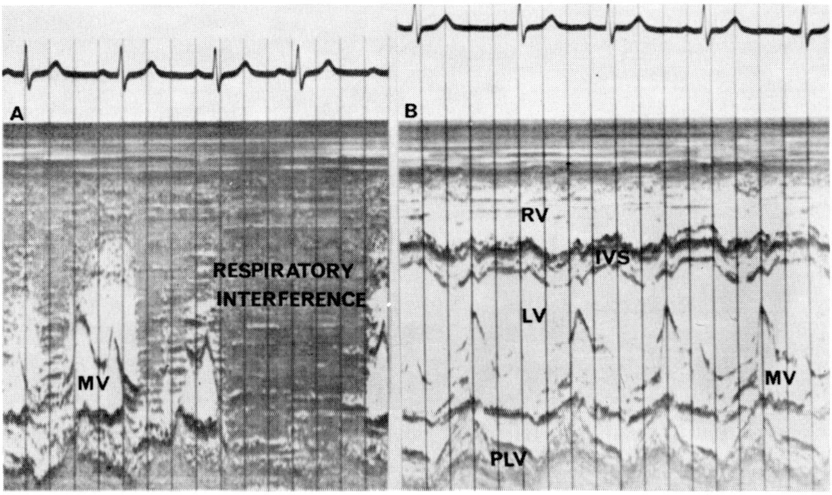

Figure 81. *A*, Transducer was positioned along left sternal border in third intercostal space to obtain tracing which is diagnostically useless because of respiratory interference. *B*, Transducer was repositioned to fourth intercostal space to obtain useful left ventricular study. RV = right ventricle, LV = left ventricle, IVS = interventricular septum, PLV = posterior left ventricular wall and MV=mitral valve.

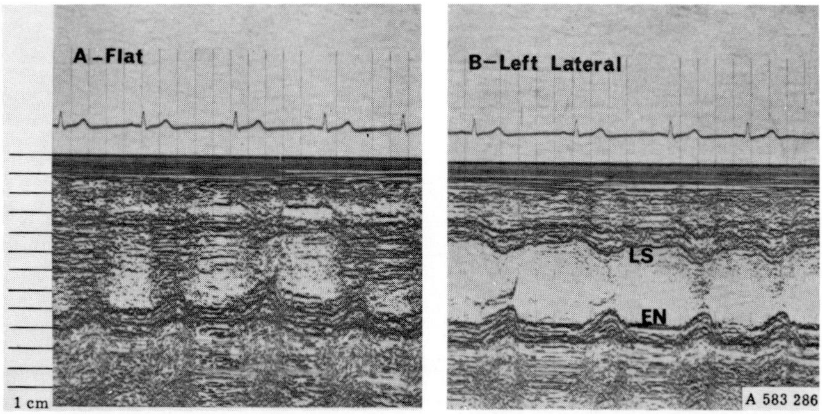

Figure 82. *A*, Left ventricular tracing obtained with patient supine; *B*, same patient, turned left laterally to obtain a more accurate left ventricular study. Transducer was placed in same intercostal space as tracing *A*. Coarse gain was decreased. LS = left septum and EN = endocardial surface of posterior left ventricular wall.

If the patient's position is altered to left lateral, a second pillow placed behind his back to maintain this position and the bed elevated approximately 20°, the heart can be rotated slightly clockwise and shifted laterally as the lung is displaced. This position places the septum and posterior wall in a more perpendicular plane in relation to the ultrasound beam; thus the septum and posterior wall are much more easily recorded (Figure 82*B*).

In some patients excessive rotation occurs, and the right ventricular dimensions will change from normal to abnormal. Any time that the examiner is considering right ventricular enlargement, the measurement of the right ventricular dimension must be taken with the patient supine.

Recording the septum and posterior wall together is probably the most time-consuming part of the echocardiographic examination. If an adequate septum is not obtainable from the transducer position originally chosen, the probe should be shifted toward the sternum and angled slightly more inferiorly and laterally. If the septum is still incomplete, the transducer should be moved upward to a higher intercostal space and angled more laterally and inferiorly.

Nearly all patients turned slightly left laterally are easier to examine. This cannot be emphasized too often. The examiner must be willing to change both patient and transducer position, depending on the patient.

Once the septum and posterior wall have been identified, it is time to make some instrumentational changes to improve the graphic appearance of the tracing:

1. The near gain control should be turned to the "off" position.
2. The depth compensation (TCG) should be set so that the slope or

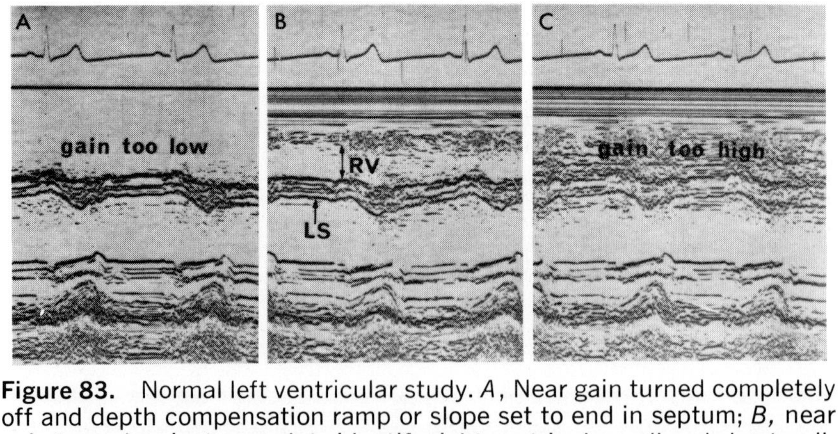

Figure 83. Normal left ventricular study. *A*, Near gain turned completely off and depth compensation ramp or slope set to end in septum; *B*, near gain turned on just enough to identify right ventricular wall and chest wall; *C*, near gain turned too high; right ventricular wall cannot be identified. RV = right ventricle and LS = left septum.

ramp *ends* in the right septum. No echoes should be seen between the right side of the septum and the transducer (Figure 83*A*).

3. Near gain may now be turned "on" just enough for the chest wall and the right ventricular wall to be visualized (Figure 83*B*). If the near gain is set too high, the right ventricular wall and the right side of the septum are not easily identified (Figure 84*C*).

Depth Scale Setting

Many newcomers to echocardiography frequently misinterpret a tracing because the depth scale setting was too compressed. Figure 84*A* has been compressed too much. The left septum and the endocardium are marked. The apparent posterior wall motion of the left ventricle (EN′) is actually from reverberations and does not represent the posterior boundary of the heart.

Figure 84*B* has been set at a depth scale of 15 cm. This scale keeps all the patterns of motion in proportion to the speed of the paper, which is run at a variable speed of 10 to 50 mm/sec. For routine work the depth scale is varied from 9 to 20 cm, depending on the size of the heart being examined. The depth scale should not be expanded to less than 9 cm even on children. The echoes become too spread out across the width of the paper, and the advantages of excellent resolution are lost.

Figure 84*C* shows the linear distortion that begins to appear when the depth scale has been spread almost entirely across the paper. While

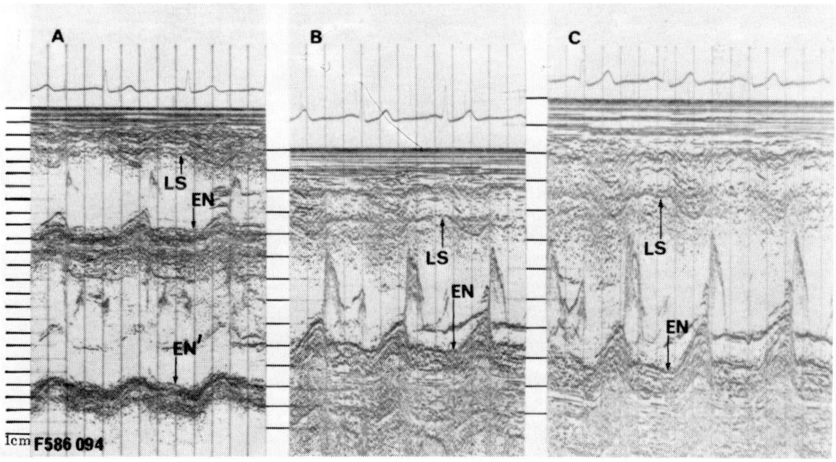

Figure 84. Patient, age 44, with lupus erythematosus and moderately severe mitral insufficiency. *A*, Tracing too compressed; *B*, proper depth setting, observing rule of fourths; *C*, tracing shows beginnings of linear distortion as depth scale becomes too spread out. LS = left septum, EN = endocardial surface of the posterior left ventricle, and EN′ = reverberation from true posterior wall (EN).

the tracing is not difficult to read in this particular patient, over-expanded pediatric tracings become virtually impossible to interpret.

I like to follow a rule of fourths; on paper 6 inches wide, the top one-fourth is for the electro- and phonocardiogram and pulse if these parameters are desired; the middle one-half for the echogram; the bottom one-fourth for lung. This bottom one-fourth is not necessarily wasted paper. Frequently one scans from a normal left ventricle to a very dilated left atrium, as with mitral stenosis or insufficiency. If the echogram occupied the bottom one-fourth of the paper, the posterior left atrial wall would drop off the oscilloscope and not be seen. The tracing would have to be calibrated and the depth scale changed, all which is a nuisance.

Routine Scan

A routine scan contains four areas which have been numbered in Figure 85 for identification and description. They include 1.) area of the left ventricular study where right and left ventricular dimensions are measured; 2.) base of the heart; 3.) atrioventricular junction and lower left atrium; and 4.) high left atrium and aorta.

For the sake of consistency from one study to another, routine left and right ventricular dimensions should always be taken from area 1. Dimensions from area 2 may be wider than those from area 1 and are not as reproducible.

Notice the amplitude and direction of septal motion in area 1 as compared to area 2. In area 2 the septum does not appear to be moving vigorously. Since the transducer is being tilted toward the left atrium and aorta, it is normal for the septum to move less, even passively or paradoxically in this area.

Area 3 is at the atrioventricular junction. Left ventricular dimension, amplitude of septal motion and posterior wall motion should not be evaluated in this area.

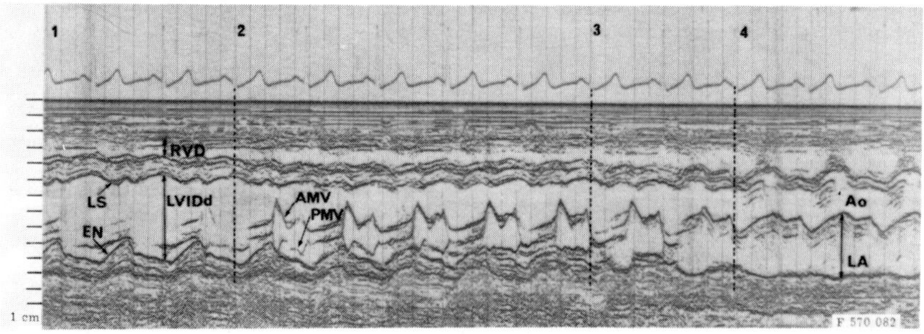

Figure 85. Routine scan from area in left ventricle below mitral valve to aorta. LS = left septum, EN = endocardial surface of posterior left ventricular wall, RVD=right ventricular dimension, LVIDd=left ventricular internal dimension during diastole, AMV=anterior mitral valve, PMV= posterior mitral valve, Ao=aorta and LA=left atrium.

By tilting the transducer higher toward the throat and rocking it slightly medial toward the right shoulder, the septum is seen to attenuate and gradually change into the anterior wall of the aorta. The posterior leaflet of the mitral valve drops out; the atrioventricular junction (area 3) gradually becomes the lower left atrial wall, which moves away from the transducer with the onset of systole. As the probe is angled even more superiorly and markedly toward the right shoulder, the passive wall of the left atrium comes into view and portions of the aortic leaflets are seen. Routine left atrial dimensions are taken from area 4.

Although we are considering the study of the left ventricle at this time, the important relationship of the ventricle to the aorta will be discussed in detail subsequently. Sometime during the average left ventricular study, scans are made to the aorta as part of our evaluation.

Pericardial Effusion

Mild Effusion

Pericardial effusion is no problem *if* the examiner follows all the rules for obtaining an accurate left ventricular study. If the effusion is present, it will show up at the time that the "damping" or "attenuation"

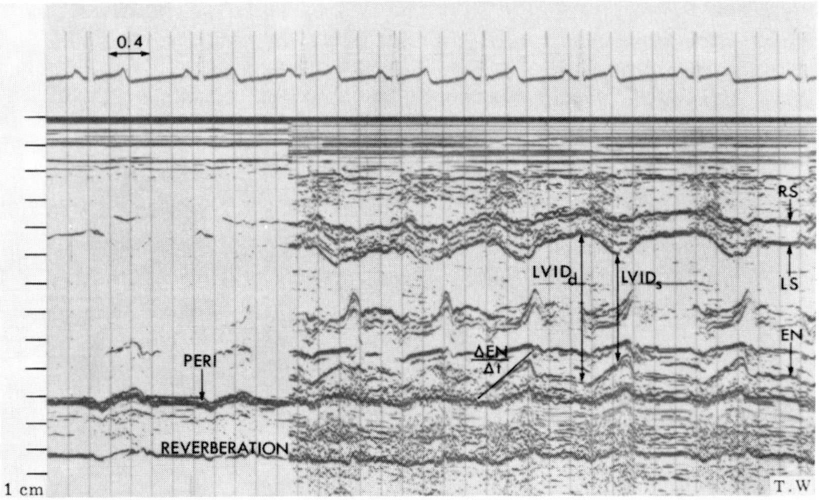

Figure 86. Normal left ventricular study. Damping has been increased at left of tracing to isolate pericardium from other posterior myocardial structures. RS = right septum, LS = left septum, EN = endocardial surface of posterior left ventricular wall, $LVID_d$ = left ventricular dimension during diastole, $LVID_s$ = left ventricular dimension during systole, peri = pericardium, $\frac{\Delta EN}{\Delta t}$ = change in endocardial amplitude divided by change in time.

is increased. One should approach every possible effusion study with the attitude that it will not be found. Obtain a routine left ventricular study, as in Figure 86, in which the septum, mitral leaflets and posterior left ventricular wall are clearly identified. When the damping is increased, the pericardium and epicardium show little or no separation from each other.

When pericardial effusions are present, there is a variable amount of separation between the epicardium and the pericardium of the left ventricle. With the small or mild effusions, it is better to "damp" the tracing or turn the "coarse gain" down to eliminate some of the stronger echoes around these structures. The effusion remains as a clear area behind the posterior wall (Figure 87).

The transducer should *never* be pointed medially when pericardial effusions are being sought. If the examiner must point the probe medially to find the septum, the patient should be turned to a left lateral position. This will rotate the heart out from under the sternum, and the septum and posterior wall will be in a more perpendicular plane to the ultrasound beam.

Moderate Effusion

As the quantity of effusion increases, so does the distance between the pericardium and the epicardium. Unless the gain is turned very low, few effusions appear to be perfectly clear. Most of them seem to be echo-producing even at low gain settings.

Figure 88 is a tracing from a 3-year-old child. Most of the fluid is seen posterior to the left ventricle. Shortly after the tracing was taken, 200 cc of fluid was tapped.

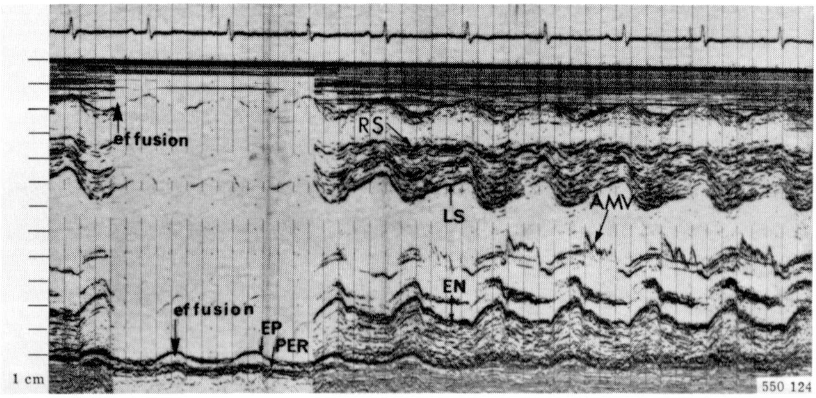

Figure 87. Female patient, age 67, with clinical diagnosis of hypertension, severe aortic insufficiency and left ventricular failure. Small pericardial effusions are very common in patients with left ventricular failure. EP = epicardium, PER = pericardium, RS = right side of septum, LS = left side of septum, EN = endocardial surface of posterior left ventricular wall and AMV = anterior mitral valve.

It is very hard to measure the volume of pericardial effusions. The tracing from Figure 88 would be read as a moderate pericardial effusion. The same criteria would fit the measurement of an effusion in an adult: there must be continuous separation of the pericardium from the left ventricular epicardium; if the quantity of the effusion is great enough, separation of the right ventricular wall from the chest wall will also be seen. Regardless of whether the patient is a child or an

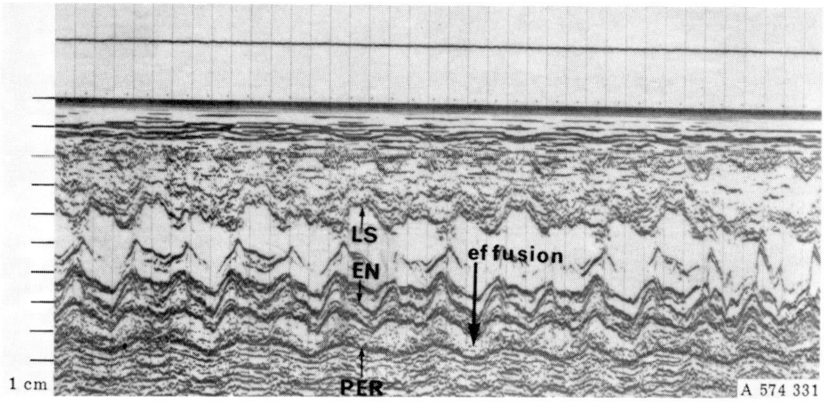

Figure 88. Child, age 3 years, referred for pericardectomy. Pericardium is separated from epicardium by 9 mm, and effusion is markedly echo-producing. Separation of right ventricular wall from chest wall is not appreciated. At surgical intervention pericardium was found to contain roughly 250 cc of organized blood. LS = left septum, EN = endocardial surface of posterior left ventricle and PER = pericardium.

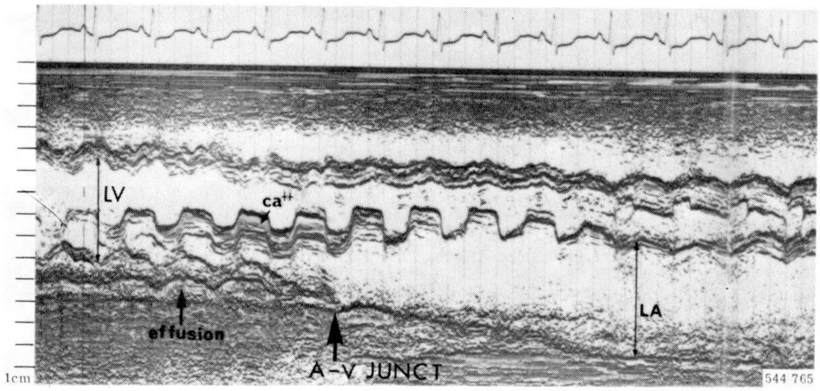

Figure 89. Female patient, age 46, with severe calcific mitral stenosis and moderate mitral insufficiency. Epicardium separates from pericardium approximately 6 mm during diastole. Effusion is localized behind posterior left ventricle and phases out at atrioventricular junction during scan from left ventricle to left atrium and aorta. LV = left ventricle, ca^{++} = calcium, A-V JUNCT = atrioventricular junction and LA = left atrium.

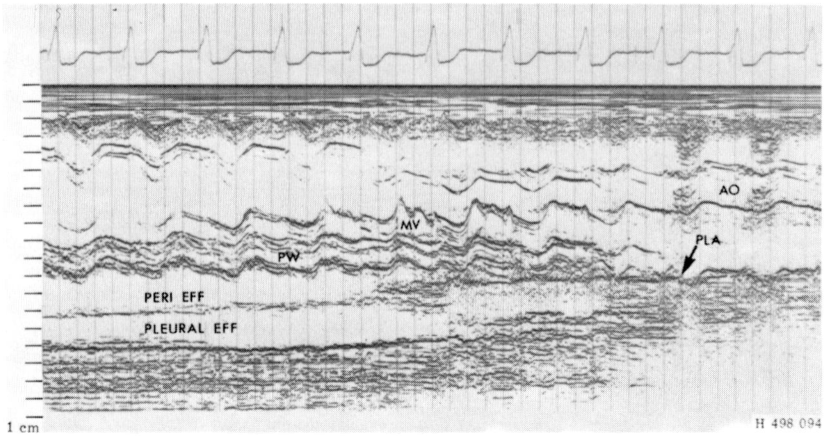

Figure 90. Female patient, age 72, with moderate pericardial effusion and pleural effusion. Scan from left ventricle to aorta shows pericardial effusion to phase out before posterior left atrial wall is recorded. Pleural effusion continues to be seen. PW = posterior wall of left ventricle, MV = mitral valve, AO = aorta, PLA = posterior left atrial wall, PERI EFF = pericardial effusion and PLEURAL EFF = pleural effusion.

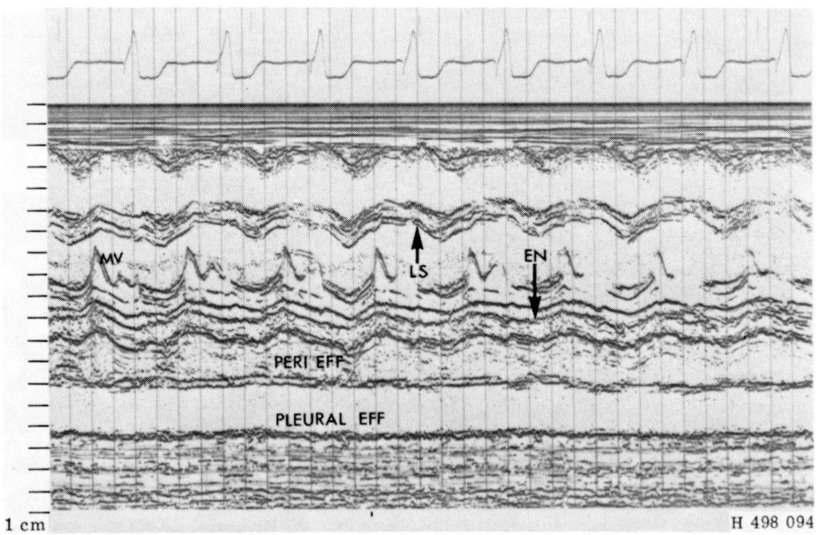

Figure 91. Same patient as in Figure 90. Transducer was repositioned to higher intercostal space to obtain more acceptable left ventricular study. There is separation between chest wall and right ventricle, indicative of anterior pericardial effusion. There is a 17-mm separation between left ventricular epicardium and pericardium. Left ventricular dimension measures 4.1 cm, right ventricular dimension measures 2.4 cm and septal motion is abnormal, owing to pacemaker and pericardial effusion. MV = mitral valve, LS = left septum, EN = endocardial surface of posterior left ventricular wall, PERI EFF = pericardial effusion and PLEURAL EFF = pleural effusion.

adult, moderate effusions appear similar on the echogram. Only the quantity of fluid is different.

Another method to determine if the examiner is dealing with a pericardial or a pleural effusion is to tilt the transducer toward the left atrium while the paper records continuously during the scan. If pericardial effusion is present, the effusion will phase out as the left atrium is approached (Figure 89). Because the pulmonary veins insert at the level of the atrioventricular junction, there is no communication between left ventricle and left atrium at the level of the pericardium. Thus pericardial effusion is trapped at the level of the atrioventricular junction.

No Pericardial Effusion

Figure 92 shows a very large pleural effusion but no pericardial effusion. Notice that there is no separation between the epicardium and the pericardium. As the transducer is tilted toward the left atrium, the posterior wall shows normal transition into the left atrial wall. The large echo-free space (pleural effusion) is seen continuously under the left atrium. Respiration is causing some interference and should not be read as echo-producing fluid. By observing these characteristics, we know that we are not pointing medial and picking up mediastinal structures, creating a "false" effusion. All the criteria for an accurate left ventricular study have been fulfilled.

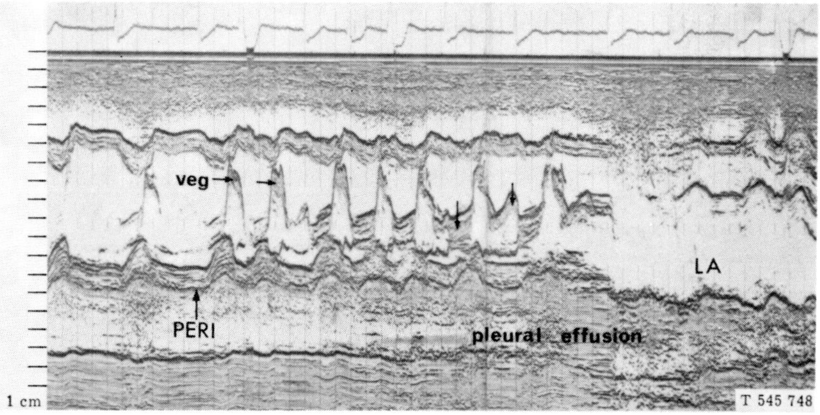

Figure 92. Male patient, age 63, with severe mitral insufficiency and severe congestive heart failure, prior to mitral valve replacement. Description of mitral valve at operation is noted in the text for Figure 23. There was no pericardial effusion seen at operation. There was a very large amount of pleural fluid which was removed by aspiration. PERI = pericardium, veg = vegetations and LA = left atrium.

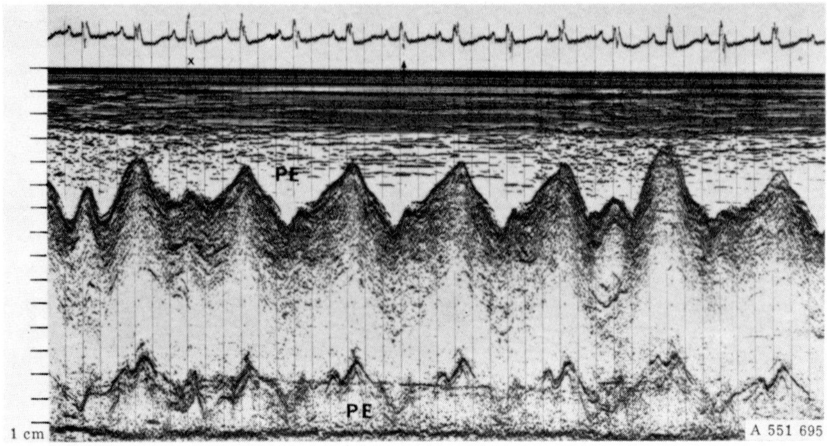

Figure 93. Massive pericardial effusion, volume estimated at 1000 cc±300 cc. The small (x) and (↑) marking the electrocardiogram indicate electrical alternans. PE = pericardial effusion.

Large Effusion

Massive effusions are easy to identify. The most striking feature is the grossly moving structure (right ventricular wall) separated by a very large space from the chest wall (Figures 93 and 94). A somewhat damped but similarly moving echo moves posteriorly and is separated from the pericardium by an echo-free space. This is the so-called swinging heart in which only the front and back walls of the heart are easily seen. The echo-free spaces are fluid filled, usually bloody and malignant. The volume of pericardial fluid may be 800 to 2000 cc in an adult. Septal and mitral valve structures may be recorded by repositioning the transducer to a higher intercostal space. *No attempt to measure ventricular dimensions or evaluate septal or valvular motion should be made until some fluid has been removed.*

Left Ventricular Volume Overload

Exaggerated septal motion and posterior left ventricular wall motion are characteristic in left ventricular volume overloaded states such as aortic insufficiency (Figure 95), mitral insufficiency, patent ductus and ventricular septal defects.

If the volume overload has been sufficiently long standing, the left ventricular dimension will dilate beyond normal limits. In aortic insufficiency the mitral valve usually flutters. It is unusual to see the mitral valve flutter in mitral insufficiency, although we have seen some do this. Catheterization-proven cases of pure, massive mitral insufficiency show echocardiograms with mitral valves moving abnormally during diastole, but the characteristic flutter seen with aortic

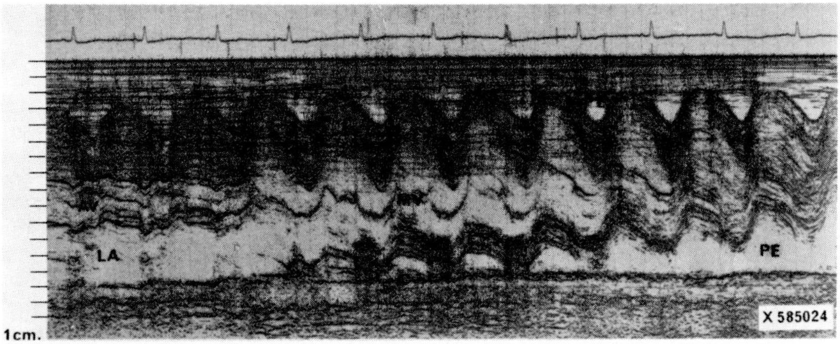

Figure 94. Female patient, age 78, with history of chronic pericarditis, referred for evaluation of status of aortic valve. Routine scan from aorta toward apex of left ventricle. Pericardial effusion is seen posteriorly just as atrioventricular junction is passed and increases in quantity as apex is approached. AV = aortic valve, LA = left atrium, MV = mitral valve and PE = pericardial effusion. (From Bonner, A., *et al.*: An unusual precordial pulse and sound associated with large pericardial effusion. Chest, in press.)

insufficiency is modified. The anterior leaflet may move chaotically rather than respond with fine vibrations. Mitral fluttering with ventricular septal defects has been reported in children.

To calculate the velocity of circumferential fiber shortening as an indication of muscle contractility, a number of formulas are in the literature. The formula used at this laboratory is:

$$VCF = \frac{LVID_d - LVID_s/ET}{LVID_d}$$

We have found a more reliable indicator of decreasing left ventricular function in the progressive dilatation of the base of the left ventricle. In studies recently completed the velocity of circumferential fiber shortening (VCF) was variable in serial studies on the same patient and did not indicate the reduced ventricular function as reflected in the patient's symptoms.

Right Ventricular Volume Overload

Figure 96 was taken from a patient with primary pulmonary hypertension and a small right-to-left shunt at the atrial level. The septum moves toward the transducer at the peak of the R wave on the electrocardiogram (dotted line), then moves posteriorly shortly thereafter. This is a variant from normal but the significance has not been worked out in any individual study.

All echocardiographic studies involving suspected dilated right ventricles must be done with the patient supine. Some normal individuals have had normal right ventricular dimensions in the supine

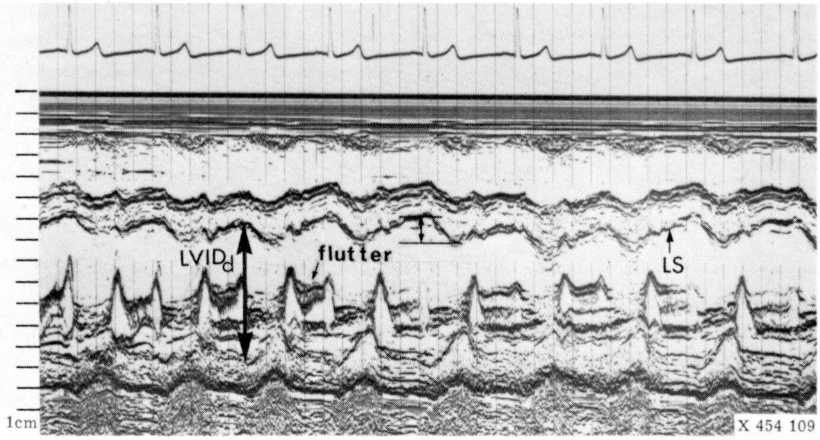

Figure 95. Male, age 18, with aortic insufficiency, possibly owing to bicuspid aortic valve. Tracing exhibits classic left ventricular volume overload features of exaggerated septal and posterior wall motion, dilated left ventricle and gross fluttering of mitral valve. LS = left septum and $LVID_d$ = left ventricular internal dimension during diastole.

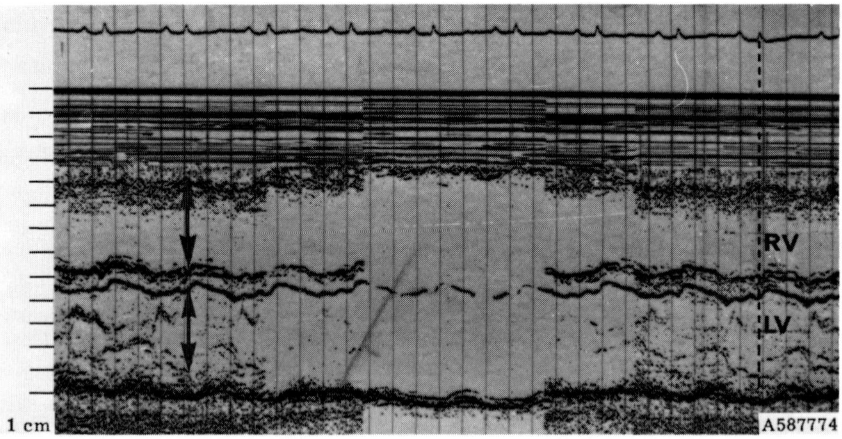

Figure 96. Diabetic female patient, age 41, with primary pulmonary hypertension and small right-to-left shunt. Pulmonary artery pressure was 75/42 mm Hg with a mean of 46 mm Hg. Resting cardiac output was 4.4 L/min with an index of 2.5 L/min/M^2. Pulmonary vascular resistance was elevated at 13.6 units. RV = right ventricle and LV = left ventricle.

position, but they became grossly abnormal when the subject turned to a left lateral position. The reason for this change in normal subjects is thought to be attributable to excessive rotation of the heart when they turn on their left side. Therefore, to eliminate this source of possible error when evaluating a patient with suspected right ventricular volume overloads, the right ventricular dimension should be taken from tracings recorded in the flat position.

Atypical Septal Motion

When the right ventricle pumps more blood than the left ventricle, the former becomes dilated. In addition, the septum moves paradoxically or becomes flattened. Atrial septal defects, tricuspid insufficiency, anomalous venous return or pulmonary insufficiency may cause both the septum to move abnormally and the right ventricle to dilate.

However, when pericardial effusion is present the septal motion may be changed from the type of motion expected. Figure 97 demonstrates this variation of septal motion. At catheterization the pulmonary artery pressure was 35/7 mm Hg with a mean of 20 mm Hg. There was a 3.1 : 1 left-to-right shunt at the atrial level. Despite the large size of the atrial septal defect, the septum's only abnormal motion is a slight anterior motion toward the transducer at the peak of the R wave on the electrocardiogram.

Paradoxical Septal Motion

The size of the right ventricle is not an accurate indicator of the size of the atrial septal defect. Figure 98 is from a patient with a small shunt, only 1.5 : 1 left-to-right, of the secundum type. Mean pulmonary artery pressure was 34 mm Hg.

The right ventricle is nearly as large as the left ventricle. The septum moves toward the transducer at the peak of the R wave on the electrocardiogram. This anterior motion is termed "paradoxical" and is indicative of right ventricular volume overload *if* accompanied by a dilated right ventricle.

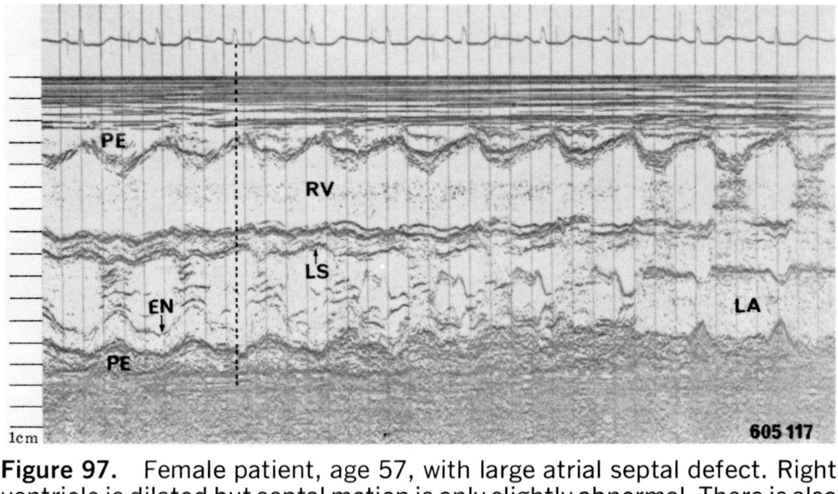

Figure 97. Female patient, age 57, with large atrial septal defect. Right ventricle is dilated but septal motion is only slightly abnormal. There is also moderate pericardial effusion. PE = pericardial effusion, EN = endocardial surface of posterior left ventricular wall, RV = right ventricle, LS = left septum and LA = left atrium.

With Left Ventricular Volume Overload

The right ventricular dimension of Figure 99 is grossly dilated at 4.8 cm. The septal motion is slightly anteriorly moving at the peak of the R wave on the electrocardiogram; the septum then immediately moves posteriorly away from the transducer. The septal motion is not truly paradoxical as it is in Figure 98.

At catheterization an atrial septal defect with a shunt flow ratio of 3.6:1 was demonstrated. Mean pulmonary artery pressure was 30 mm

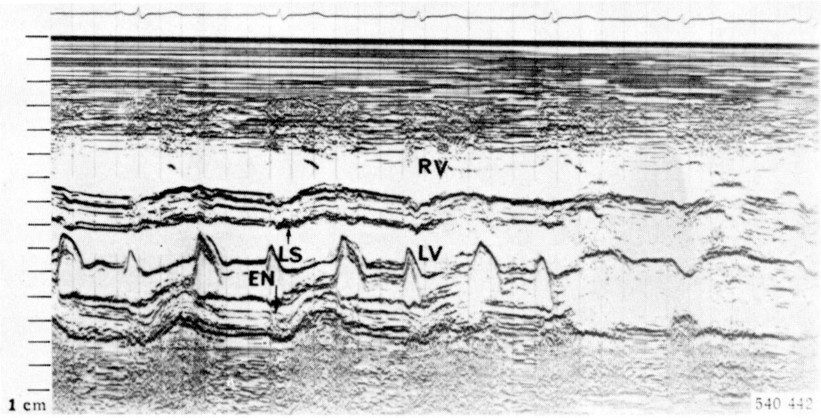

Figure 98. Female patient, age 52, with small atrial septal defect of secundum type. RV = right ventricle, LV = left ventricle, LS = left septum and EN = endocardium.

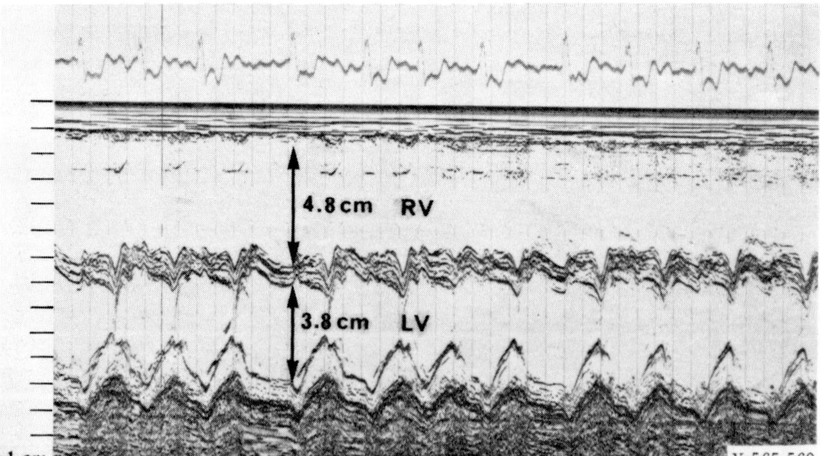

Figure 99. Male patient, age 34, referred for evaluation of heart murmur. There was an atrial septal defect with large left-to-right shunt, with moderate mitral insufficiency. Because of very large shunt and dilution of dye, possibility of primum defect could not be completely excluded. RV = right ventricle and LV = left ventricle.

Hg. An associated finding was moderate mitral insufficiency—a left ventricular volume overload which is causing the septum to respond to the overload on the left rather than on the right.

Left Ventricular Hypertrophy

An acceptable left ventricular study showing both sides of the septum and posterior left ventricular wall with both mitral cusps should be obtained. Hypertrophy or thickening of the left ventricle may be expected in patients with severe aortic stenosis, chronic untreated hypertension, idiopathic hypertrophic subaortic stenosis and many renal diseases.

Figure 100 is taken from a patient with chronic untreated hypertension and aortic insufficiency. The thickness of the septum and of the posterior wall should be measured during diastole at the peak of the R wave on the electrocardiogram. The thickness of the septum is measured from the right to the left side, and the posterior wall is measured from endocardium to epicardium.

The normal range of thickness for a symmetrical left ventricle is 0.8 to 1.1 cm for both septum and posterior wall. Any thickness greater than 1.1 cm is considered to be hypertrophy.

In IHSS, the septum may be considerably thicker than the posterior wall. However, we have seen patients with normal septums and very thick posterior walls.

Figure 101 shows a typical case of IHSS. The septum is considerably thicker than the posterior left ventricular wall. This finding per se, however, does not automatically mean that IHSS is present. The

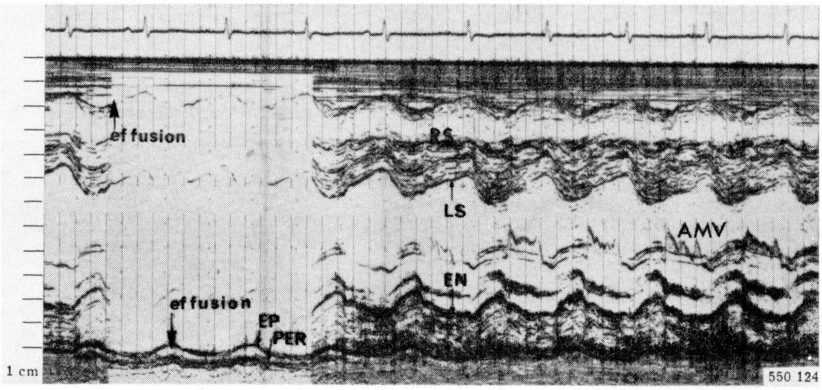

Figure 100. Patient with severe aortic insufficiency and hypertension. Her blood pressure ranged from 160/110 to 240/100 mm Hg. Left ventricular dimension is approximately 5.7 cm, posterior wall thickness of 1.9 cm, septal wall thickness of 1.3 cm and mild pericardial effusion. EP = epicardium, PER = pericardium, RS = right septum, LS = left septum, EN = endocardial surface of posterior left ventricular wall and AMV = anterior mitral valve.

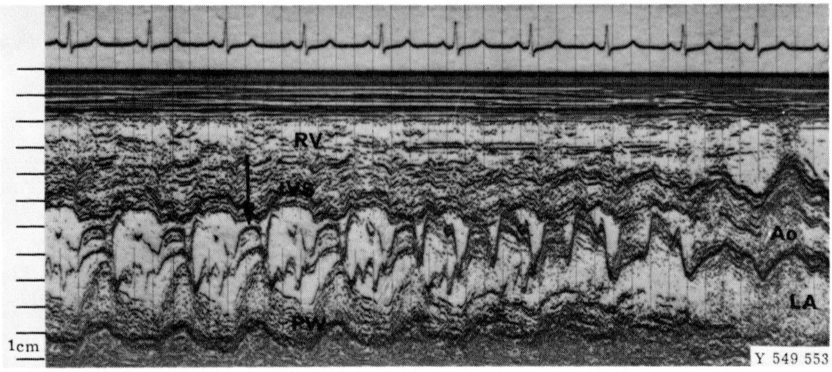

Figure 101. Patient, age 27, who had presenting symptom of murmur and family history of two children dying of hypertrophic myopathy. Additional study of family members disclosed that his father had IHSS. Scan from left ventricle to left atrium shows markedly thickened septum and mitral valve obstructing left ventricular outflow tract. RV = right ventricle, IVS = interventricular septum, PW = posterior wall, Ao = aorta and LA = left atrium.

systolic motion of the mitral valve determines the obstructive manifestations of this disease, and even that motion must be provoked at times.

Variations

Some angle compensations have to be made for those patients in whom it is difficult to locate structures according to the established procedure. Tall, thin patients with vertical hearts have septums lying in a plane almost parallel to the ultrasound beam. They should be turned to an extremely left lateral position on a flat bed.

Obese patients usually have horizontally positioned hearts. The transducer will have to be tilted more medially than usual to find the aorta and more laterally than usual to find the posterior wall. Very often the septum displays abnormal motion without dilated right ventricles. This abnormal motion may be an artifact attributable to the position at which the septum lies in relation to the sound beam.

In persons with aortic stenosis it is very difficult to record the aortic valve. By moving the transducer nearer the apex and angling in the usual plane, the valve motion may be recorded. Often the valve may be recorded from the subxiphoid position. Patients with mitral stenosis tend to have more vertically than horizontally positioned hearts. The best recording of the posterior wall is found by tilting the transducer more inferiorly. The septum is usually located under the sternum, so the patient should be turned left laterally.

Huge right ventricles obscure a clearly delineated left ventricular study. The patient should be rolled to his *right* to rotate the heart toward a more normal position; the left ventricular dimension should be easier to obtain. To obtain the right ventricular dimension, the patient should be returned to the supine position.

Septums that cannot be found at all are usually under the sternum. The patient should be rolled to the left lateral position and the transducer position adjusted by moving it closer to the sternum or up one or two intercostal spaces. Difficult mitral valves may be obtained as the patient is brought toward a sitting position. It is reported that prolapsed mitral valves are also easier to obtain by this method.

Condensed M-Mode Scanning

Left Ventricle

In an effort to obtain an overview of the heart, the paper speed of the strip chart recorder was slowed to 10 mm/sec rather than the routine 25 to 50 mm/sec. The angle of the transducer was slowly and constantly altered from the aorta to the apex while recording was continued (Figure 102).

By condensation (or compression) of a normal scan, the left ventricle appears to taper to a smaller dimension as the apex is approached. The motion of the septum and of the posterior wall seems exaggerated, although this is an optical illusion. If the amplitude of motion were to be measured, the examiner would find the values to be the same as those recorded at faster speeds. The apparent exaggeration of wall

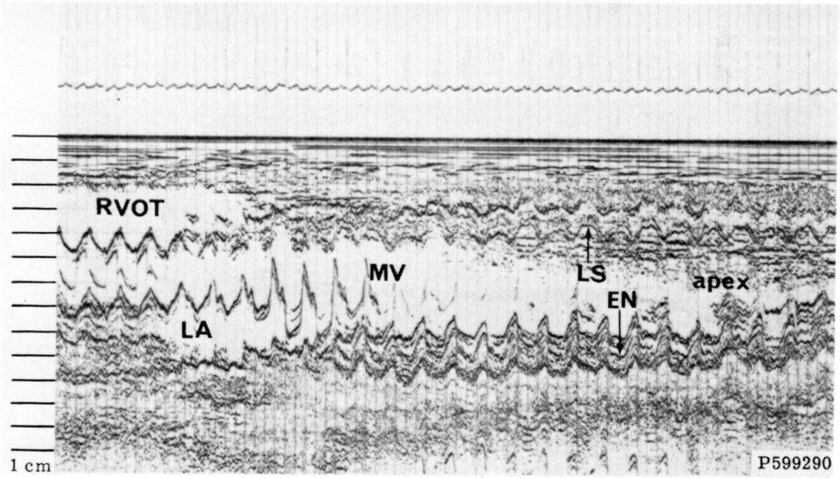

Figure 102. Condensed scan from patient with normal left ventricle. Effect of tapering as apex is approached is consistent with symmetrically shaped left ventricle as seen during cineangiography in absence of left ventricular dysfunction. RVOT = right ventricular outflow tract, LA = left atrium, MV = mitral valve, LS = left septum and EN = endocardial surface of posterior left ventricular wall.

motion allows the examiner to appreciate subtle changes occurring in wall motion as the sound beam transects different areas of the heart throughout the scan. Many of these changes cannot be appreciated at faster recording speeds without considerable measuring. At slow recording speeds these changes are evident at a glance.

Once recording of the condensed scan has begun, the examiner must be careful to keep the transducer moving in a smooth and constant motion. The beam should transect a different part of the heart every time the heart beats.

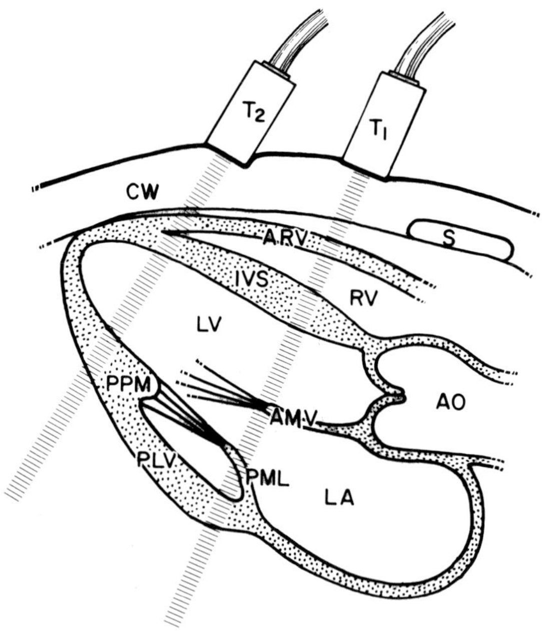

Figure 103. Standard placement of transducer over heart for routine study of mitral valve, base of heart and aorta and left atrium (T_1). By moving transducer one intercostal space lower to position T_2 apical dimensions and wall motions may be recorded. CW = chest wall, PPM = posterior papillary muscle, LV = left ventricle, ARV = anterior right ventricular wall, RV = right ventricle, AMV = anterior mitral valve, PML = posterior mitral leaflet, LA = left atrium, AO = aorta, S = sternum, PLV = posterior left ventricular wall and IVS = interventricular septum.

Does it make any difference which intercostal space is used to examine the heart? If the transducer was placed in position T_1 (Figure 103) and angled toward the apex, the sound beam would be oblique to the posterior wall at the level of the papillary muscles. The apical dimension would appear to be markedly dilated and the posterior wall would not move well. To place the sound beam most perpendicular to the walls of the apex at the level of the posterior papillary muscle, the transducer is moved one intercostal space lower (Figure 103 T_2) and slightly laterally.

Figures 104, 105 and 106 were recorded from the same patient with the transducer placed in three different intercostal spaces. Routine right and left ventricular dimensions and left atrial dimension are commonly taken from the type of tracing depicted in Figure 105, since the transducer is most centrally located in relation to the base of the heart.

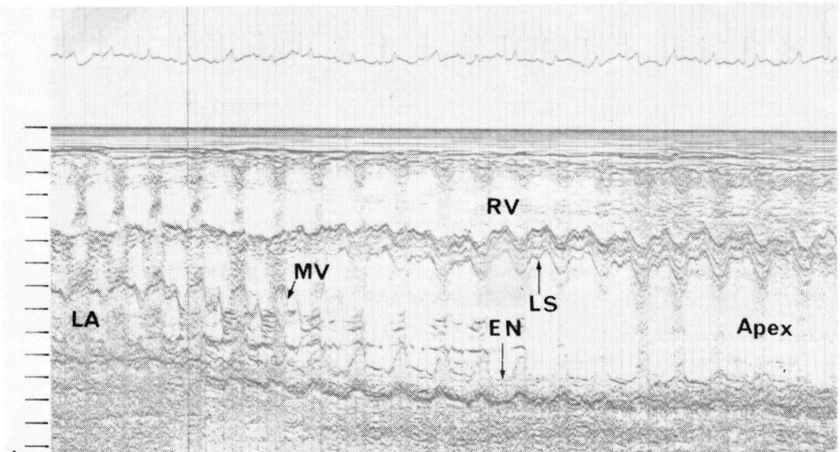

Figure 104. Scan from aortic area toward apex, transducer located in second intercostal space. Aortic area is not clearly defined. As transducer is tipped inferiorly toward mitral valve, multiple echoes are recorded from anterior leaflet during systole; they should not be interpreted as thickened valve. As transducer is tipped further inferiorly toward apex, septum remains intact and becomes exaggerated in amplitude during systole. Posterior wall amplitude appears to decrease and may be misinterpreted as segmental disease. Apical wall motions should not be evaluated from this position. LA = left atrium, MV = mitral valve, LS = left septum, EN = endocardial surface of posterior left ventricular wall and RV = right ventricle.

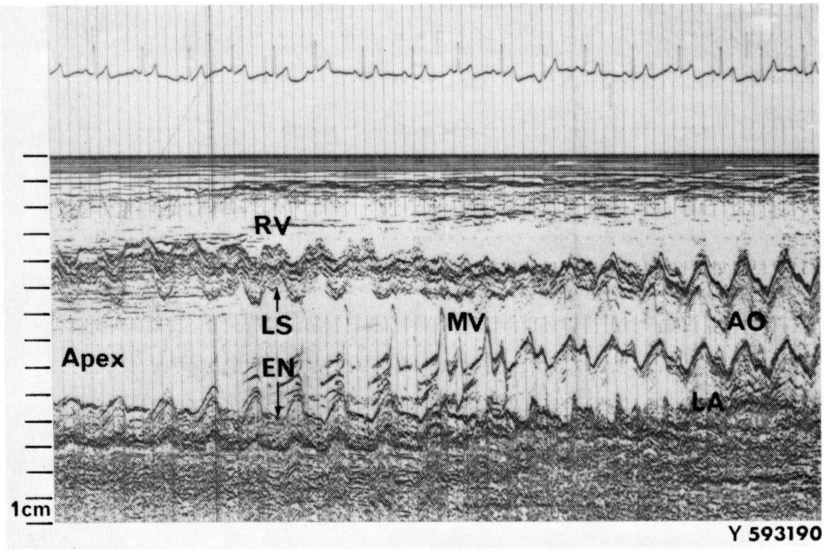

Figure 105. Scan from apex to aorta, with transducer positioned in third intercostal space. Transducer is approximately central in relation to heart's position in chest. Mitral valve lies fairly perpendicular to sound beam. By tilting transducer equal distances toward aorta or apex, structures remain well defined. This is area from which usual dimensions, wall thicknesses, amplitude of wall motion and examination for pericardial effusion are obtained. RV = right ventricle, MV = mitral valve, AO = aorta, LA = left atrium, LS = left septum and EN = endocardial surface of posterior left ventricular wall. (From Chang, S., Feigenbaum, H., and Dillon, J.: Condensed M-mode echocardiographic scan of the symmetrical left ventricle. Chest 68:93, 1975.)

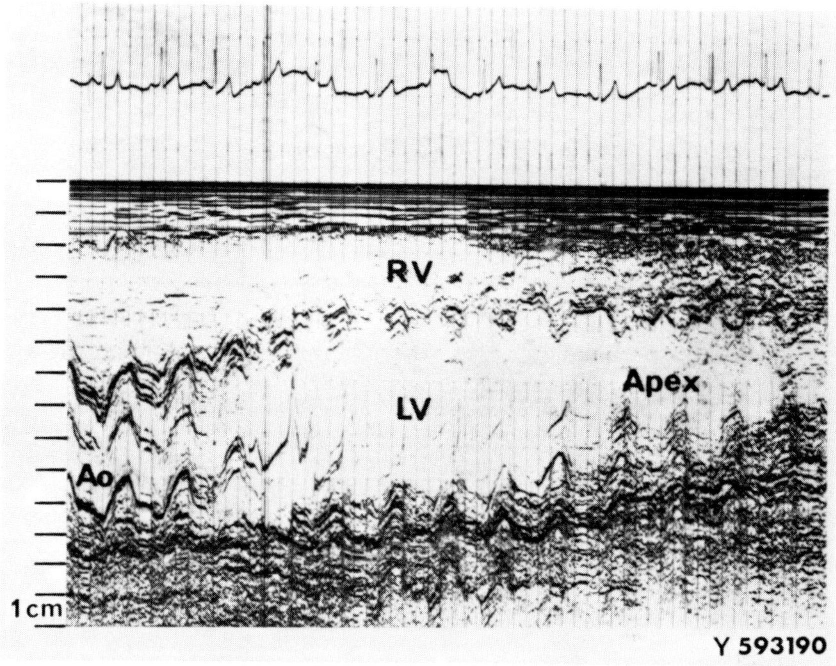

Figure 106. Scan from aorta to apex, with transducer repositioned to fourth intercostal space. Sound beam is now low in relation to heart's position in chest. Beam is also more perpendicular to walls near apex at level of posterior papillary muscles. Apical left ventricular dimension may be measured. One should not attempt to obtain basilar left ventricular dimensions from tracing taken this close to apex. Ultrasound beam is oblique to high septum, which causes it to be broken and poorly defined. Ao = aorta, RV = right ventricle and LV = left ventricle. (From Chang, S., Feigenbaum, H., and Dillon, J.: Condensed M-mode echocardiograph scan of the symmetrical left ventricle. Chest *68*:93, 1975.)

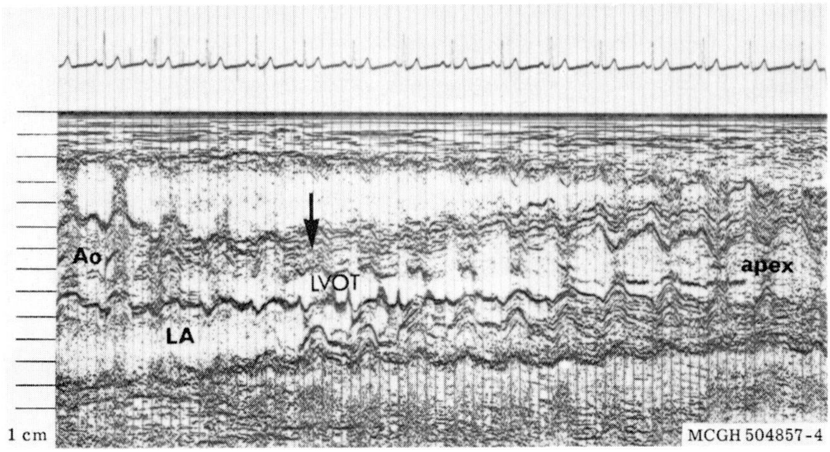

Figure 107. Female patient, age 58, with catheterization-proven IHSS. There was no resting subaortic gradient and no gradients following premature ventricular beats except on one isolated occasion in which gradient of 26 mm Hg was noted. After Valsalva maneuver, 14 mm Hg gradient was obtained and after amyl nitrite stimulation, gradient increased to 48 mm Hg. Isoproterenol stimulation produced marked gradient of 139 mm Hg. Cineangiography demonstrated mild aortic insufficiency. Ao=aorta, LA=left atrium and LVOT=left ventricular outflow tract.

Idiopathic Hypertrophic Subaortic Stenosis (IHSS)

The transducer was positioned superiorly toward the aorta and then gradually angled inferiorly and laterally toward the apex while the paper was recording at 10 mm/sec. The fourth intercostal space was the only position that could be used for adequate studies.

The septum is thickened in the area of the high mitral valve (Figure 107, arrow). Normal motion and thickness are evident in the area of the apex. Bulging of the mitral valve is not apparent during systole and suggests no significant left ventricular outflow obstruction with rest.

Discrete Subaortic Stenosis

The transducer was angled from the deep ventricle toward the aorta and left atrium (Figure 108). The systolic bulging of the mitral valve appears somewhat atypical, and gross fluttering of the mitral valve indicates significant aortic insufficiency. The septum is not thickened as would be seen with muscular subaortic stenosis. Instead there is an additional echo-producing interface (Figure 108, arrow), which is the diaphragmatic band obstructing the left ventricular outflow tract.

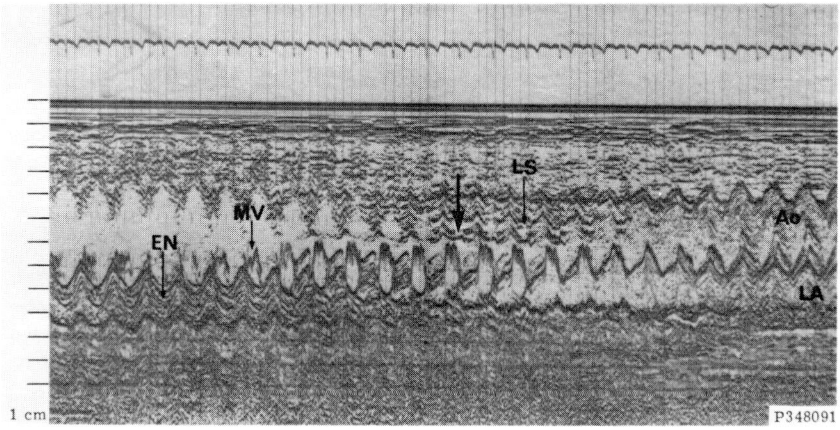

Figure 108. Female patient, age 17, with catheterization-proven discrete subaortic stenosis. Gradient across left ventricular outflow tract measured 75 mm Hg. Moderately severe aortic insufficiency was also demonstrated by cineangiography. MV = mitral valve, LS = left septum, Ao = aorta, LA = left atrium and EN = endocardial surface of posterior left ventricular wall.

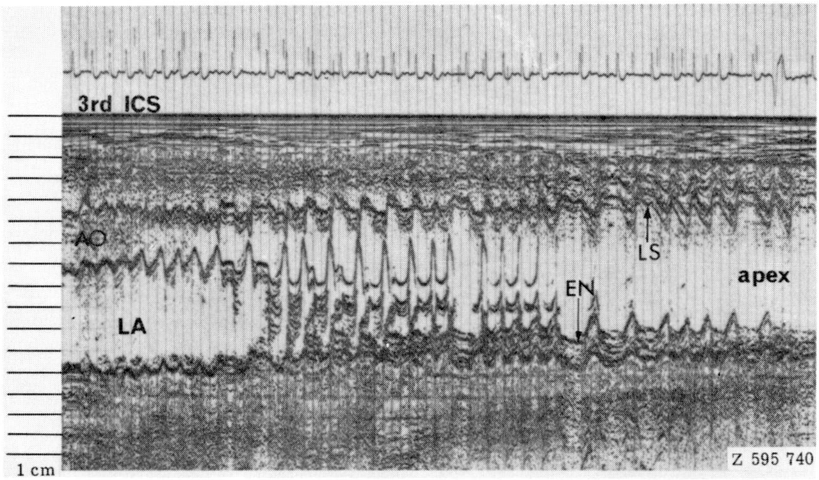

Figure 109. Female patient, age 48, with catheterization-proven severe mitral insufficiency. Deterioration was significant during previous five years. During that period cardiac output was normal. At present, cardiac output has decreased significantly. Patient's pulmonary vascular resistance was elevated at four units at rest and 3.3 units with exercise. LA = left atrium, AO = aorta, LS = left septum and EN = endocardial surface of posterior left ventricular wall.

Mitral Insufficiency

Figure 109 was recorded from the third intercostal space, the scan being from the aorta toward the apex. The left ventricular dimension is dilated, and the septum moves with exaggerated motion. The posterior left ventricular wall appears to move more vigorously in the area of the low mitral valve and then to lessen as the transducer is directed toward the apex.

Figure 110 was obtained by repositioning the transducer to the fourth intercostal space more laterally so that the beam was directed through the apex at the level of the papillary muscles. The area of apex which did not appear to move well from the third intercostal space (Figure 109) then moved normally. The dimension of the apex is dilated, and one would expect the heart to be globular. This was borne out by cineangiographic examination.

Myopathy

Unlike the tracings from Figures 109 and 110, the posterior wall motion of Figures 111 and 112 appears to be reduced from both intercostal spaces. The apical septal motion seems to be somewhat better from the fourth intercostal space. This tracing was taken from a teenage male in whom the presenting symptoms were of myocarditis, probably of viral origin. This type of tracing from a much older patient

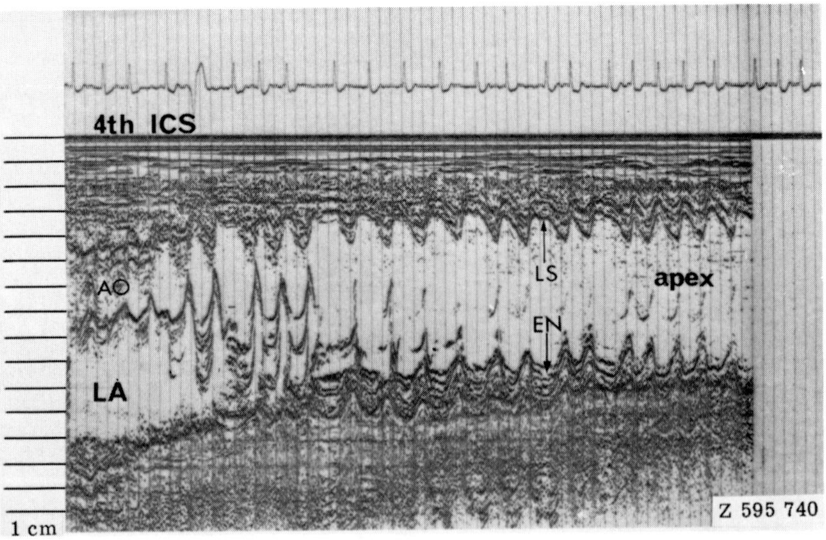

Figure 110. Same patient as in Figure 109. Scans from two different intercostal spaces allow examiner to obtain dimensions from base of heart and apex, as well as to evaluate ventricular wall motion. This patient has severe mitral insufficiency. LA = left atrium, AO = aorta, LS = left septum, EN = endocardial surface of posterior left ventricular wall.

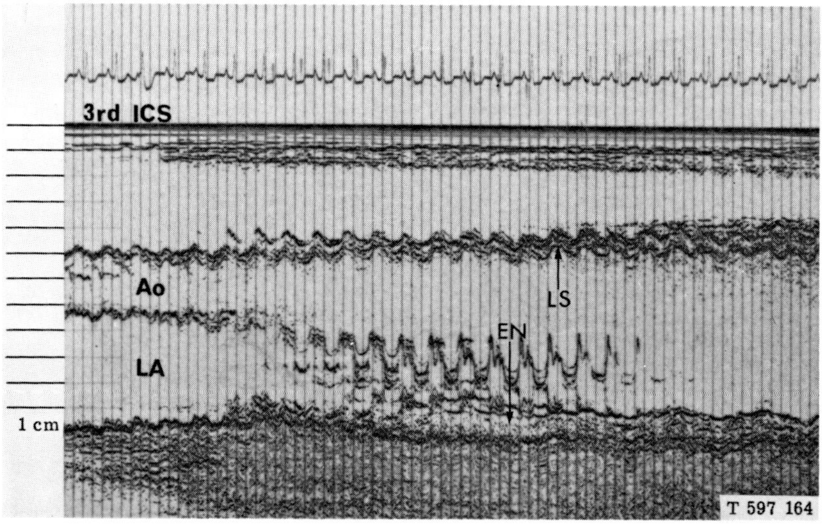

Figure 111. Scan from aorta toward apex. Septum is seen to move in normal direction but with reduced amplitude. Posterior left ventricular wall contributes very little to total effective stroke volume. Left ventricle is markedly dilated at approximately 6.5 cm. Ao = aorta, LA = left atrium, LS = left septum and EN = endocardial surface of posterior left ventricular wall.

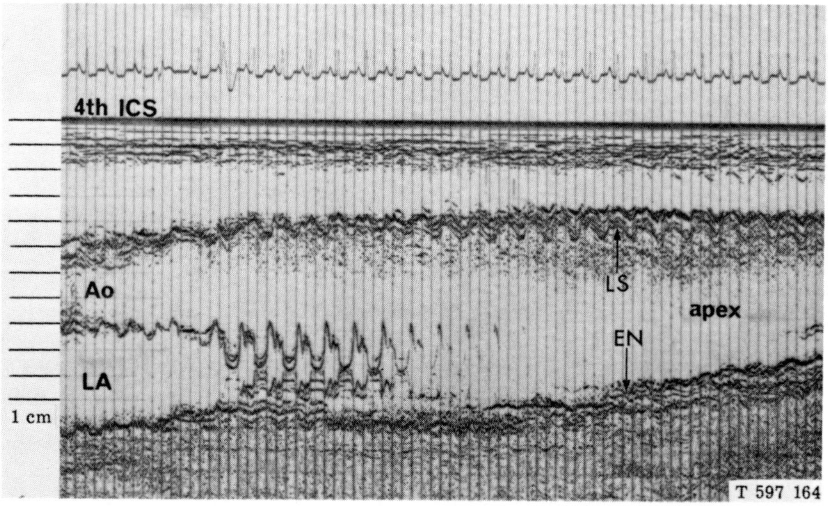

Figure 112. Scan from same patient as in Figure 111, with transducer repositioned to fourth intercostal space. Even though sound beam is perpendicular to posterior left ventricular apical wall, motion remains markedly diminished. Apical dimension is approximately 4.9 cm, which is at upper limits allowed normally. Apex seems to taper to narrower dimension. If this patient were much older, finding could just as well be interpreted as suggestive of coronary artery disease, involving posterior left ventricular wall in particular. However, this patient demonstrated myopathy. Ao = aorta, LA = left atrium, LS = left septum and EN = endocardial surface of posterior left ventricular wall.

would be very difficult to interpret. One would be tempted to suggest coronary disease based on the variability of motion between the septum and posterior left ventricular wall. It should be realized that wall motion is diffusely diminished in both severe coronary artery disease and myopathies, and the ability to distinguish between the two is not always possible.

Tetralogy of Fallot

A high membranous ventricular septal defect causes the septum to drop out of the recording as the transducer is tilted from the left ventricle to the aorta (Figure 113). The larger the defect, the clearer the area of the defect of echoes which cannot be recorded, since that part of the septum does not exist. Smaller ventricular septal defects may be missed because some tissue around the defect will be detected by moving into the sound beam and will thus be recorded. Muscular ventricular septal defects deeper in the ventricle have not been recorded at this laboratory by M-mode echocardiography.

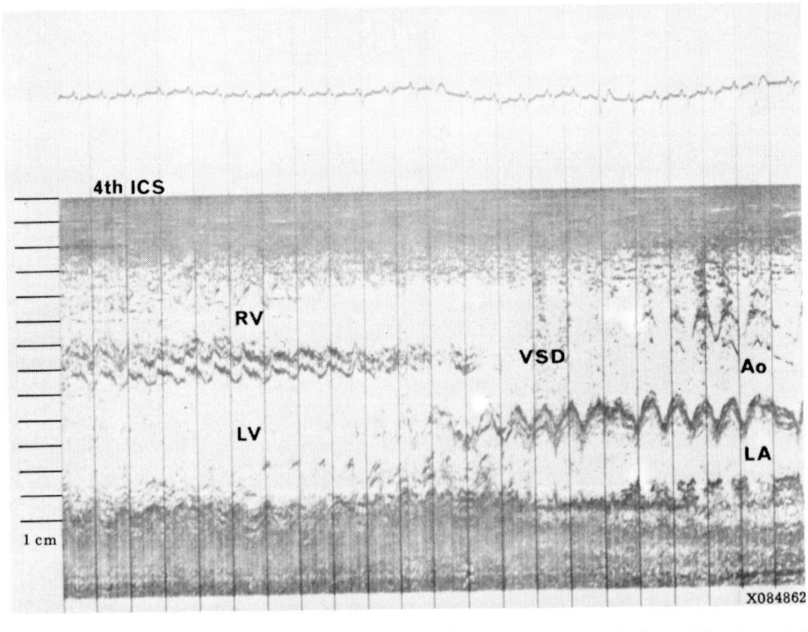

Figure 113. Patient, age 44, with proven tetralogy of Fallot. Distinguishing features on this tracing are dilated right ventricle, right ventricular wall hypertrophy and discontinuity between septum and anterior aorta. RV=right ventricle, LV=left ventricle, VSD=ventricular septal defect, Ao=aorta and LA=left atrium.

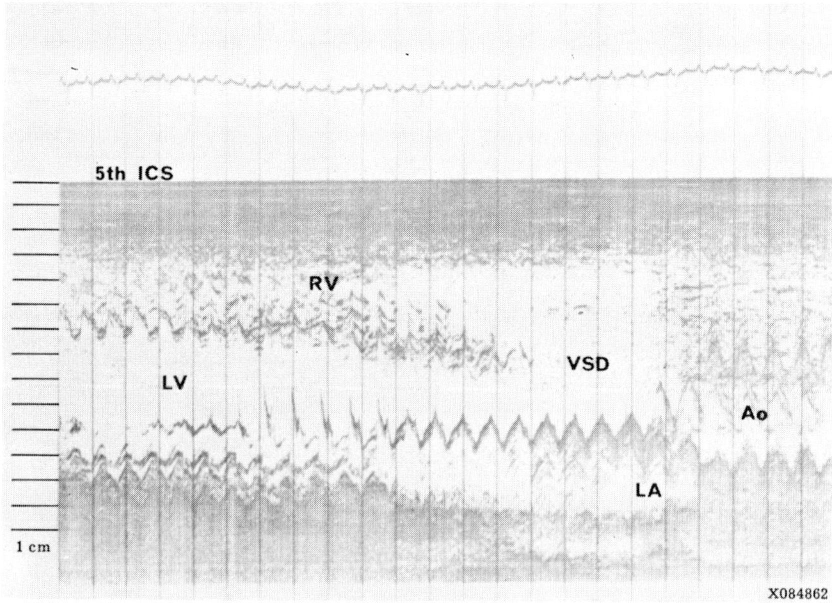

Figure 114. This scan from apex to left atrium is from same patient as in Figure 113. Discontinuity between septum and anterior aorta persists even from different examining position. Owing to absence of echoes in VSD area, defect is considered to be large. LV = left ventricle, RV = right ventricle, VSD = ventricular septal defect, LA = left atrium and Ao = aorta.

False Overriding of Aorta

The patient in Figure 115 had as a presenting symptom a marked chest deformity identified as carinatum. The transducer was placed in the second intercostal space and angled from the left ventricle superiorly to the aorta. The septum seems to disappear into the aorta, although no definite empty space can be identified as a ventricular septal defect. The aorta appears to be evenly split by the septum and overlaps both right and left ventricles.

The transducer was then moved to the third intercostal space, and a condensed scan was repeated, this time beginning from the aorta and proceeding inferiorly to the left ventricle (Figure 116). The anterior aortic wall and the septum are now seen to be intact and in their proper relationship to each other. There is no longer any suggestion of overriding of the aorta. The aortic valve appears to be thickened, as does the mitral valve which also seems to be prolapsing. The pericardial effusion and the dimension of the left atrium should not be evaluated or measured from this lower intercostal space since the tracings are not technically satisfactory for these purposes.

Any time that an overriding aorta is suspected, the examiner should record scans from multiple intercostal spaces. The effect of "overrid-

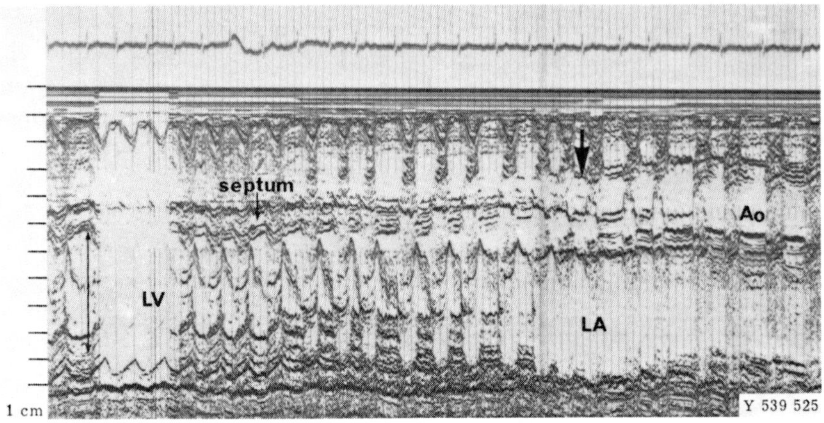

Figure 115. Patient, age 51, being echocardiographically evaluated for mitral and aortic valve disease. Transducer is placed in second intercostal space and angled from left ventricle to aorta. Aorta seems to override both ventricles although no definite ventricular septal defect can be identified. There is moderate pericardial effusion and dilated left atrium. LV = left ventricle, Ao = aorta, LA = left atrium and arrow = anterior aorta.

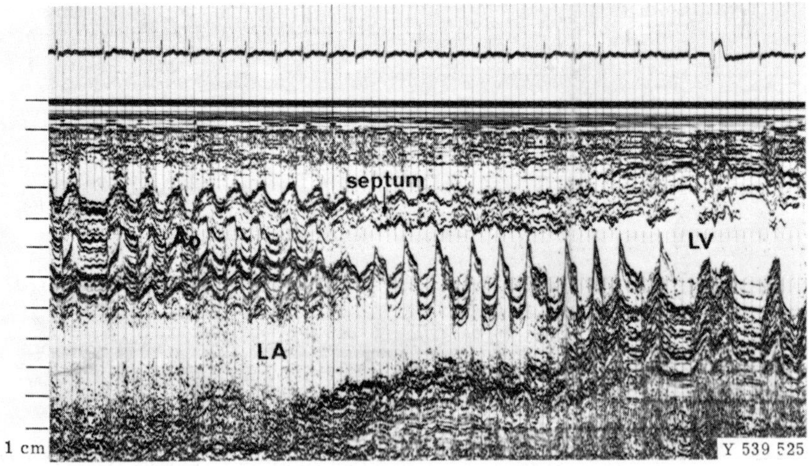

Figure 116. Scan from aorta to left ventricle, in patient with mitral insufficiency. Unlike tracing taken from second intercostal space showing "overriding aorta," tracing from third intercostal space shows complete continuity between anterior aorta and septum. Multiple scans in this area did not suggest membranous ventricular septal defect. Ao = aorta, LA = left atrium and LV = left ventricle.

ing aorta" in Figure 115 was manufactured by having the transducer positioned too high in relation to the position of the heart within the chest. Other chest deformities that may alter the position of the transducer in relation to the heart's position are "straight-back syndrome" and "pectus excavatum." False overriding of the aorta has been demonstrated in patients with these abnormalities at this laboratory.

Subxiphoid Examination

Adequate studies cannot always be obtained from along the left sternal border, and another approach to the heart must be attempted. Patients with barrel chests, emphysema or coronary artery disease are suitable candidates for a subxiphoid examination.

The transducer should be placed slightly to the right of the patient's midline and gently but firmly pressed downward and tilted superiorly toward the throat (Figures 117 and 118). The transducer should not be jabbed into the subxiphoid. This is painful for the patient and causes improper positioning of the probe.

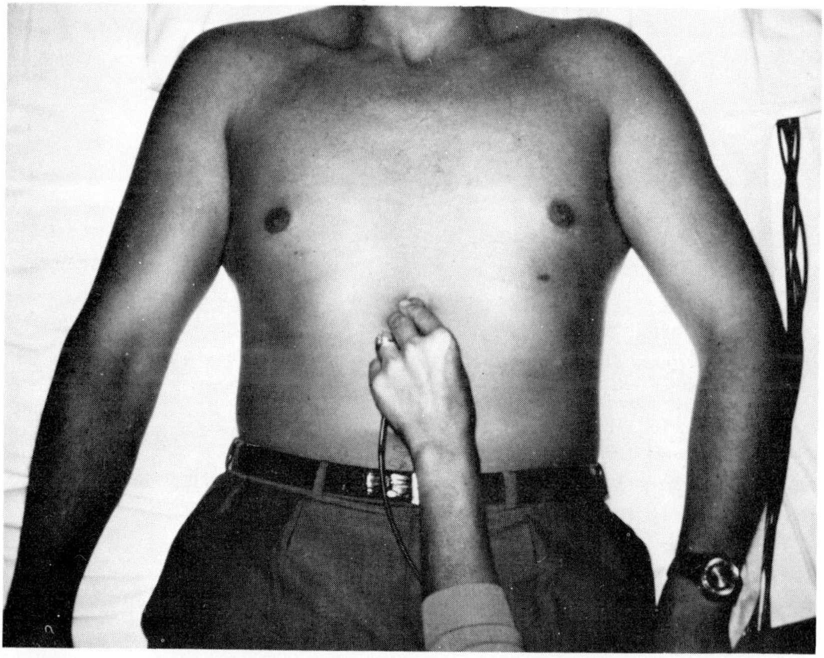

Figure 117. Placement of transducer at subxiphoid position. Most examinations are conducted with transducer positioned more to patient's right of the midline (sternum). This places sound beam more perpendicular to desired ventricular structures. (From Chang, S., and Feigenbaum, H.: Subxiphoid echocardiography. J. Clin. Ultrasound *1*:14, 1973.)

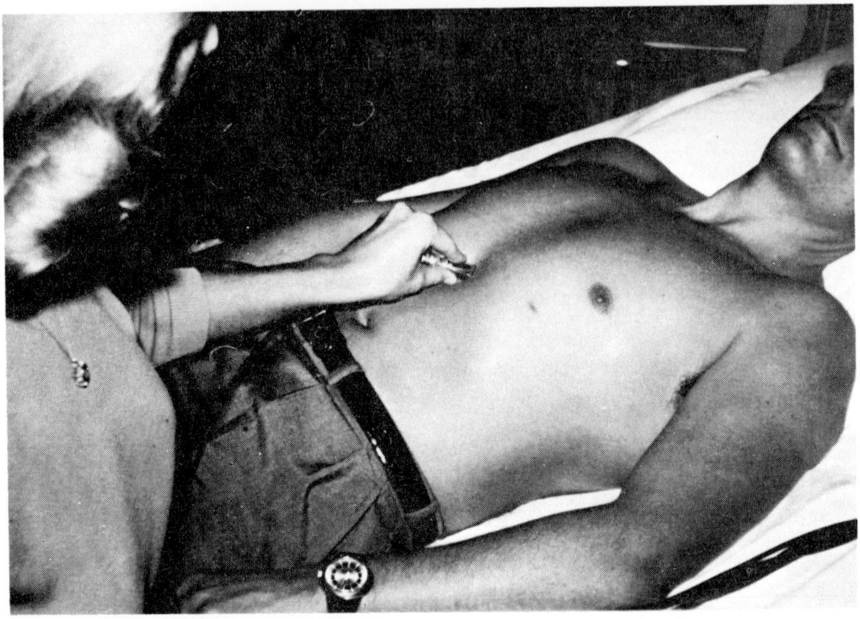

Figure 118. Side view of subxiphoid examination. Probe positioning is easier if abdominal muscles can be relaxed by elevating patient's head and torso to 20° to 30° or by having patient draw up his knees so that soles of the feet rest comfortably flat on bed.

The structures to be examined from this position now lie in a sector-scan between the tricuspid valve and the apex. Diagram C (Figure 119) shows the major structures transected, depending on the angle at which the transducer is positioned. Compare the structures recorded subxiphoid vs those recorded from the left sternal border (Figure 119*A* and *B*).

Figure 120 demonstrates the need for a subxiphoid examination. The tracing from the fifth intercostal space along the left sternal border is not adequate for measuring left ventricular dimensions. The examiner cannot be sure which structure is the septum. By repositioning the transducer subxiphoid, the septum is easily identified and valid ventricular dimensions can be obtained.

Dimensions obtained from the subxiphoid position are valid and comparable to measurements obtained from the left sternal border. The only dimension that cannot be measured is the right ventricular. The right ventricle is not a symmetrical chamber, and the examiner is never sure if the beam is transecting the belly of the right ventricle, in which case the dimension will be dilated; or if the beam is passing through the apex, in which case the dimension will be normal (Figure 121).

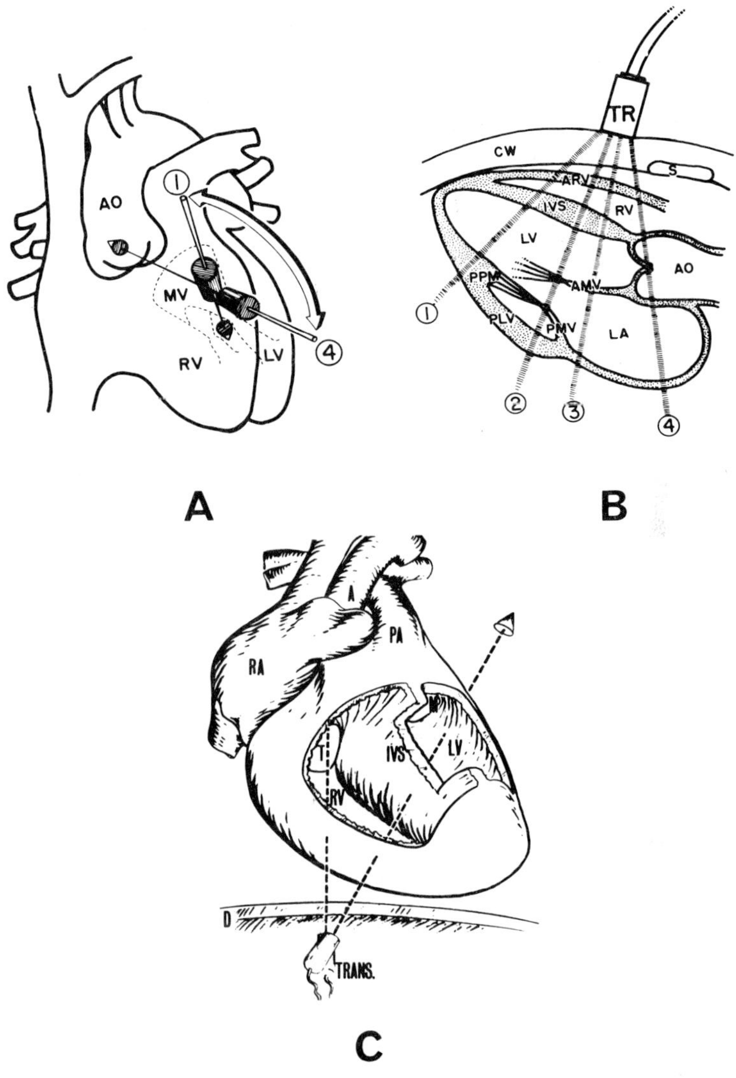

Figure 119. *A*, Transducer positioned along left sternal border and arced in sector-scan between aorta and low mitral valve; *B*, structures through which sound beam passes as transducer is arced in sector-scan between aorta and low mitral valve; *C*, structures through which sound beam passes with transducer positioned subxiphoid and arced in sector-scan between tricuspid and aortic valves to the apex of left ventricle. A and AO = aorta, MV = mitral valve, RV = right ventricle, LV = left ventricle, TR = transducer, CW = chest wall, ARV = anterior right ventricular wall, S = sternum, IVS = interventricular septum, PPM = posterior papillary muscle, PLV = posterior left ventricular wall, PMV = posterior mitral valve, AMV = anterior mitral valve, LA = left atrium, RA = right atrium, PA = pulmonary artery, T = tricuspid valve, M = mitral valve and D = diaphragm. (*A, B,* from Feigenbaum, H.: *Echocardiography,* Philadelphia, Lea & Febiger, 1972; *C,* from Chang, S., *et al.*: Subxiphoid echocardiography. J. Clin. Ultrasound *1*:14, 1973.)

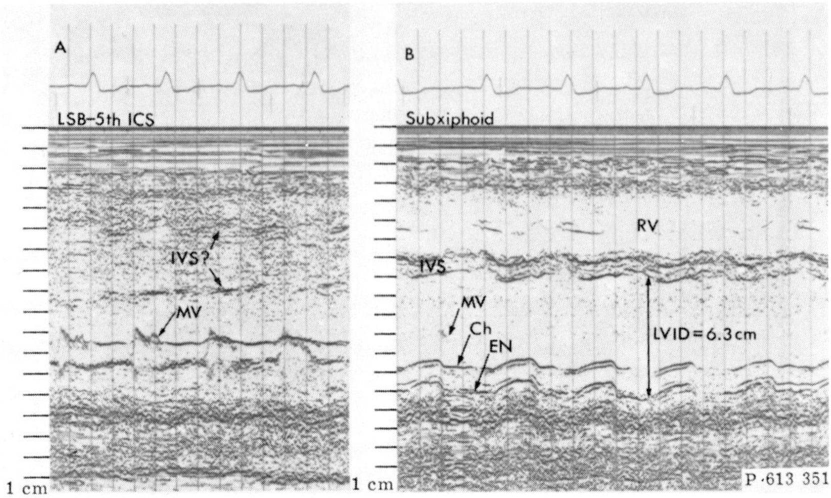

Figure 120. *A,* Technically unsatisfactory tracing of left ventricle from along left sternal border; *B,* subxiphoid tracing from same patient. Septum is now evident and left ventricular dimensions can be made and ventricular wall motion evaluated. Differential diagnosis of primary cardiomyopathy vs. "burned-out" hypertensive-ischemic heart disease with cardiomegaly has not been resolved by cardiac catheterization. Patient was advised to follow program of medical management. IVS = interventricular septum, MV = mitral valve, Ch = chordae, EN = endocardial surface of posterior left ventricular wall, RV = right ventricle, and LVID = left ventricular internal dimension during diastole.

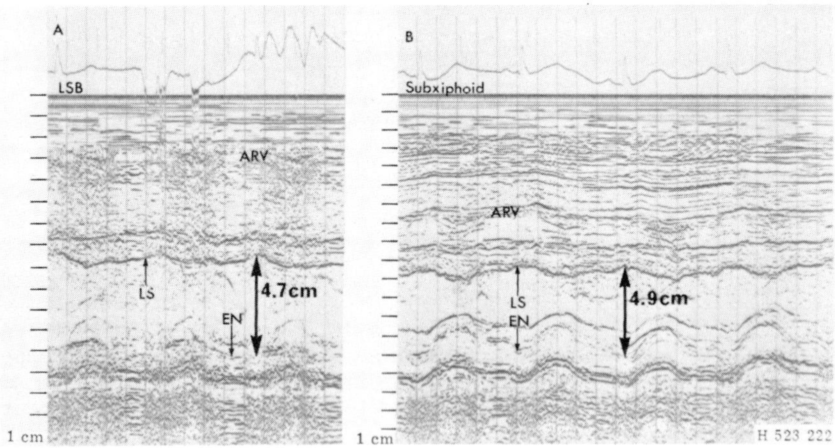

Figure 121. *A,* Tracing from along left sternal border. Technically this tracing is satisfactory for making left ventricular and right ventricular dimensions and for evaluating ventricular wall motion; *B,* for comparison a subxiphoid study was done. Ventricular dimensions are comparable; right ventricular dimension is considerably less from subxiphoid position and should not be measured. ARV = anterior right ventricular wall, LS = left septum, EN = endocardial surface of the posterior left ventricular wall and LSB = left sternal border.

Left ventricular wall thickness, wall motion, and motion of the aortic, tricuspid and mitral valves may be evaluated accurately in most cases. Pericardial effusion evaluation is comparable whether recorded through the chest or subxiphoid. The technique is especially valuable in evaluating the cardiac status in patients from whom technically unsatisfactory studies are obtained from along the left sternal border (Figure 120*A*).

Figure 122 was taken from a patient who had severe calcific aortic stenosis and mild aortic insufficiency. Selective coronary cineangiography showed normal coronary arteries. Because of the extreme reduction of septal motion, the examiner considered the possibility of left anterior descending coronary artery disease, prior to cardiac catheterization. Figure 123 was recorded from the subxiphoid position to evaluate the diaphragmatic septal motion, which was normal. Left ventricular dimensions were comparable between examination methods.

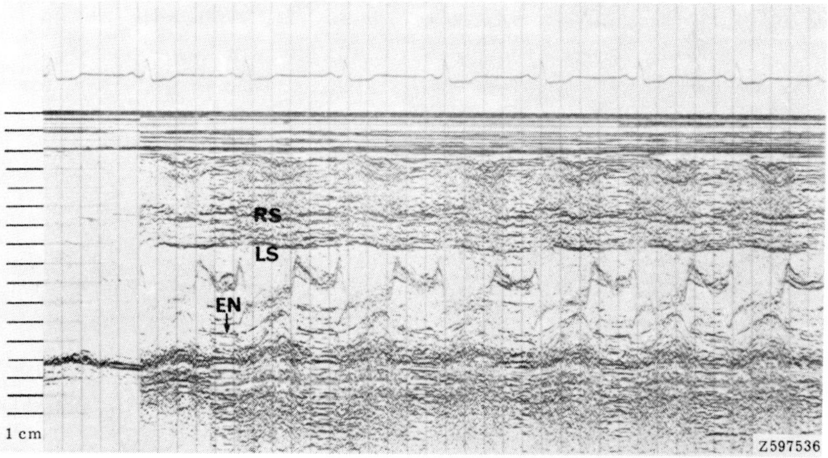

Figure 122. Male patient, age 54, with severe aortic stenosis and chronic obstructive lung disease. Poor motion of septum may be result of position of transducer to septum; or it may be owing to hypertrophy of wall. Coronary artery cineangiograms disclosed no areas of narrowing. RS = right septum, LS = left septum and EN = endocardial surface of posterior left ventricular wall.

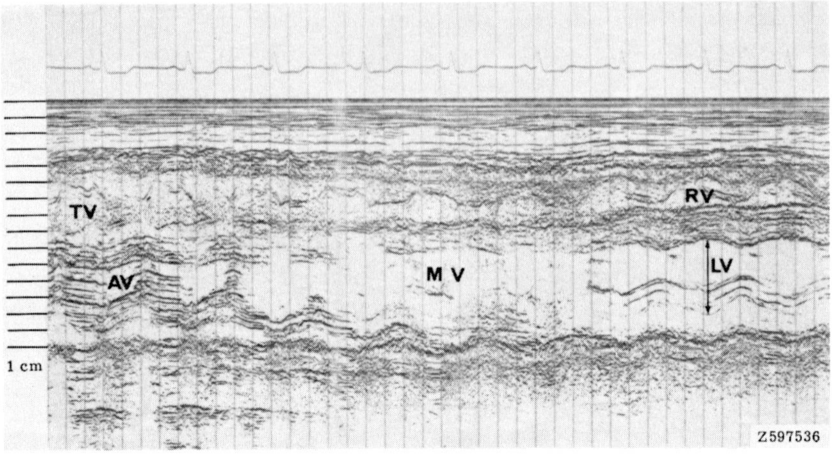

Figure 123. Subxiphoid tracing from same patient as in Figure 119. Transducer was arced in sector-scan from tricuspid-aortic valve area toward left ventricular apex. More motion is exhibited by septum from this examination site. TV = tricuspid valve, AV = aortic valve, MV = mitral valve, RV = right ventricle and LV = left ventricle.

Identification of Main Pulmonary Artery

Commonly the tricuspid and aortic valves may be recorded simultaneously from the subxiphoid position. The chamber behind the aorta had never been definitely identified until the motion of a Swan-Ganz catheter was recorded. Figure 124*A* shows the aorta with some of the leaflet structures. Posterior to the aorta is the structure designated as the catheter in the main pulmonary artery. Figure 124*B* shows the catheter in the right ventricle in the area where the tricuspid valve is usually seen, as well as in the main pulmonary artery. No studies were done to see if the diameter of the main pulmonary artery could be determined from the subxiphoid position.

Pericardial Effusion

Figure 125*A* was the best tracing obtained from the left sternal border. The septum and posterior wall are technically unacceptable. A small pericardial effusion appears to be present but should not be interpreted from such a poor tracing.

To obtain a better tracing, the transducer was positioned subxiphoid (Figure 125*B*). The septum and posterior left ventricular wall with some mitral valve are technically suitable for evaluation. Again a small posterior pericardial effusion is evident and appears to be comparable to the amount seen by the left sternal border examination.

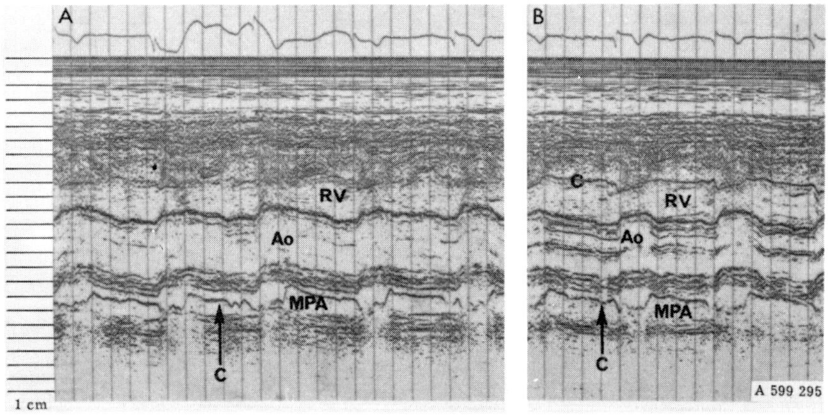

Figure 124. Male patient, age 71, with recent myocardial infarction. Swan-Ganz catheter is positioned in main pulmonary artery. RV = right ventricle, Ao = aorta, MPA = main pulmonary artery and C = catheter. (From Chang, S., Feigenbaum, H., and Dillon, J.: Subxiphoid echocardiography: A review. Chest, *68*:233, 1975.)

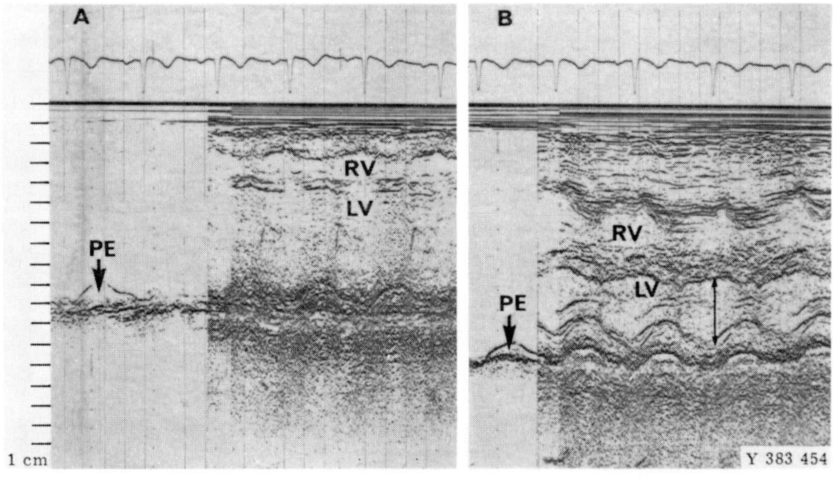

Figure 125. Female patient, age 76, referred for evaluation of "gallop." *A*, Technically unsatisfactory left ventricular study from left sternal border; *B*, technically satisfactory left ventricular study from subxiphoid position. Damping of tracing shows mild amount of pericardial effusion more clearly. RV = right ventricle, LV = left ventricle and PE = pericardial effusion.

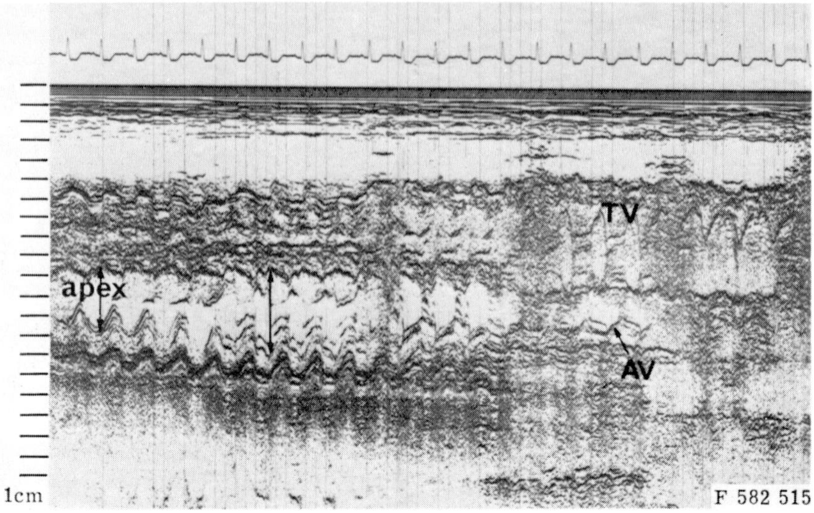

Figure 126. Female patient, age 62, with cor pulmonale and edema. Left ventricle appears to be normal at apex and base with symmetrical shape from base to apex. Recordings of 25 mm/sec were made of valvular motion. Purpose of condensed scan was to evaluate general "shape" of left ventricle. Mitral, tricuspid and aortic valves are utilized as landmarks. TV = tricuspid valve and AV = aortic valve. (From Chang, S., Feigenbaum, H., and Dillon, J.: Condensed M-mode echocardiographic scan of the symmetrical left ventricle. Chest, *68*:93, 1975.)

Normal Subxiphoid Condensed Scan

The patient from whom Figure 126 was obtained had cor pulmonale. Examination along the left sternal border was impossible. No useful echoes could be obtained from this examination site. Subxiphoid repositioning of the transducer produced technically satisfactory tracings. This condensed scan was obtained by sector-scanning from the apex to the tricuspid-aortic valve area while the paper recording speed was set at 10 mm/sec. The apex appears to be tapered, and the dimension is less than that obtained nearer the base of the heart in the mitral valve area. Septal motion and posterior left ventricular wall motion are normal.

The tracing in Figure 127 appears similar to that in Figure 126. The septum shows considerably less motion, and the dimensions of the base of the left ventricle and the apex are dilated. However, the effect of a tapered apex is still apparent.

The patient from whom this tracing was taken may have some coronary artery disease involving either the left anterior descending or the right coronary artery. It is just as possible that this patient has a myopathy; however, the posterolateral wall of the left ventricle moves too well compared to the inferior septal motion, which finding contraindicates diffuse myopathy.

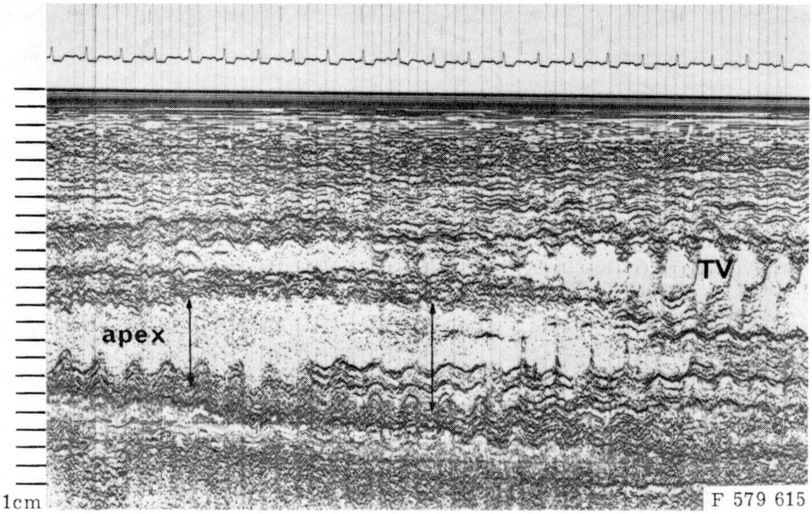

Figure 127. Male patient, age 70, referred for evaluation of an S_3 gallop, split S_1, S_4 mitral regurgitation murmur, increased shortness of breath, fatigue and congestive heart failure. Echocardiographic study was normal except for dilated left ventricle and reduced inferior septal wall motion. Pulmonary valve motion was normal elsewhere on tracing. Phonocardiogram was not helpful in clarifying diagnosis, and cardiac catheterization was not done. Tracing demonstrates some problems that examiner may have in differentiating between two diagnoses, either of which may be correct, and they may be concurrent. TV = tricuspid valve.

Coronary Artery Disease: Two Methods of Examination

Extensive information can be obtained about a patient's cardiac status by examining the heart from the left sternal border and subxiphoid. This is the standard practice followed by me in examining a patient with suspected coronary artery disease.

Figure 128 was taken from the fifth intercostal space along the left sternal border. The paper recording speed was 10 mm/sec with time-line intervals of 0.2 sec. The left side of the septum is almost indistinguishable; a left ventricular dimension from this tracing would be something of a guess at 6.8 cm. The apex is dilated.

A subxiphoid tracing was taken from the same patient recorded in Figure 128 at the same recording speed (Figure 129). The septal and posterior left ventricular walls are clearly defined, and the septal motion is seen to move abnormally. As the transducer was angled toward the apex, the dimension increased rather than tapered, as would be the case if the ventricle were symmetrically shaped.

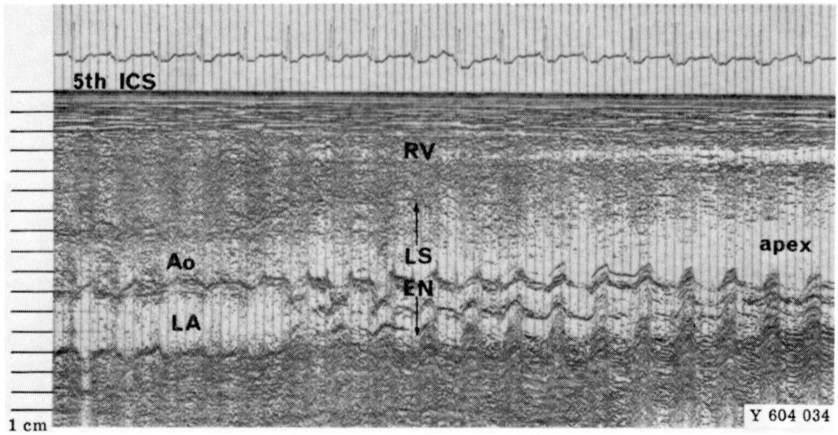

Figure 128. Condensed low scan with transducer positioned perpendicularly over apex at level of papillary muscles. Apex is dilated. Basilar dimension should not be measured since transducer is not positioned perpendicularly over mitral valve area. Tracing could not be obtained from fourth intercostal space owing to lung interference. Ao = aorta, LA = left atrium, RV = right ventricle, LS = left septum and EN = endocardial surface of posterior left ventricular wall.

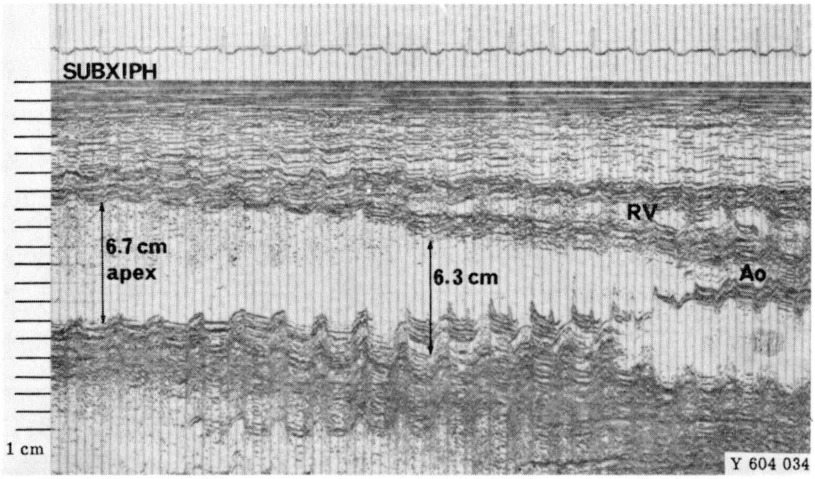

Figure 129. Condensed subxiphoid scan from 53-year-old male with catheterization-proven apical ventricular aneurysm and totally occluded left anterior descending coronary artery just distal to its origin. Sector-scan was performed by angling transducer from apex to base to aorta. Apical aneurysm was surgically resected and obstructed coronary artery was by-passed. RV = right ventricle and Ao = aorta.

Figures 130 and 131 demonstrate the need for multiple examination methods to assess left ventricular function. The routine basilar dimension could not be obtained from the third intercostal space. The low apical dimension was obtained from the fourth intercostal space. The apical anterior septal motion appears to be normal, but the septal motion in the mitral valve area is not seen well enough to evaluate (Figure 130). The posterior left ventricular wall motion in the area of the low mitral valve appears to be normal with diminishing motion toward the apex.

The tracing from the subxiphoid examination site revealed a dilated base and a tapered apex with more motion of the apical septum than was seen at the base in the mitral valve area. The right coronary artery was totally occluded in its proximal portion. It was thought that the inferior apical septum continued to move well since it was supplied by a system of collaterals that filled retrograde from the left system.

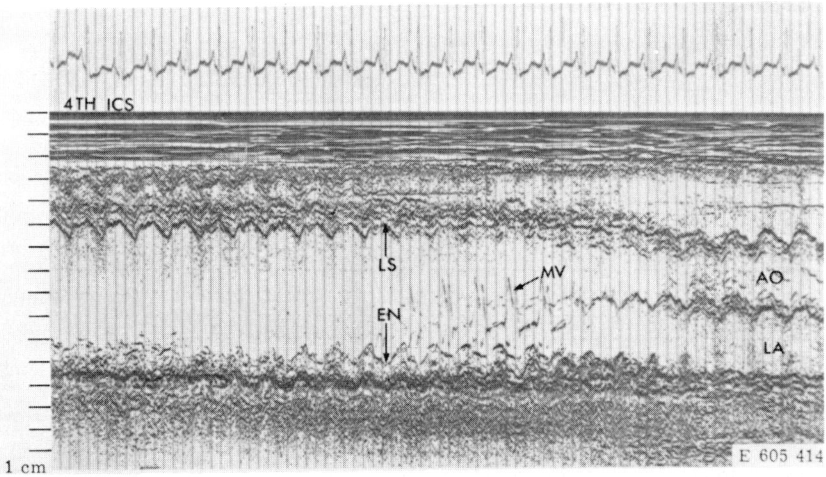

Figure 130. Male patient, age 48, with severe triple vessel coronary artery disease. Left ventriculogram revealed extensive akinesia of inferior wall and hypokinesia of anterior wall. LS = left septum, EN = endocardial surface of posterior left ventricular wall, MV = mitral valve, AO = aorta and LA = left atrium.

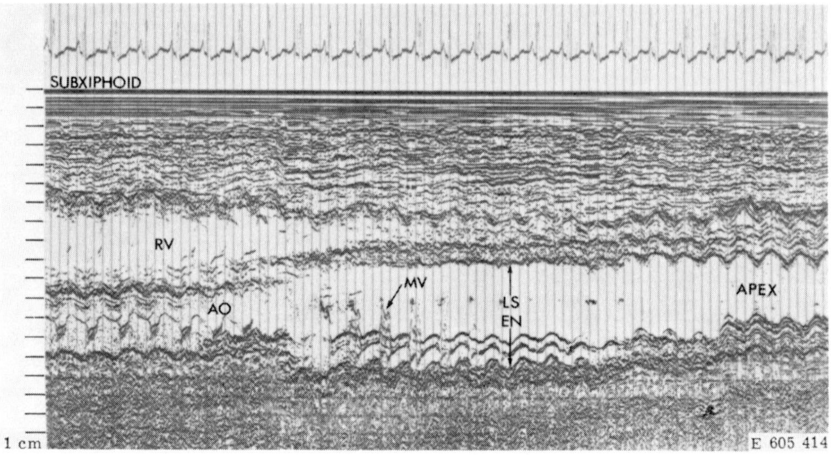

Figure 131. Subxiphoid condensed scan from same patient whose tracing is Figure 130. Sector-scan from aorta to apex discloses inferior septum with very poor motion, improving as apex is approached. Posterolateral wall motion is adequate from base to apex. Difference between apical dimension obtained subxiphoid vs one obtained from fourth intercostal space indicates some dilatation of apex in anteroposterior plane. Efficient apical wall motion suggests system of collaterals supplying apical portion of septum. RV = right ventricle, AO = aorta, MV = mitral valve, LS = left septum and EN = endocardial surface of posterolateral left ventricular wall.

Figure 132 was obtained from a 72-year-old male from the left sternal border. The position of the aortic anterior wall in relation to the left septum at the level of the mitral valve places the scan in between a mid and low examination site. The ventricle is dilated; the anterior septal motion is akinetic; the posterior wall motion is exaggerated, possibly compensating for the abnormal septal motion. Other portions of the original tracing disclosed a prolonged PR–AC interval indicative of elevated left ventricular end-diastolic pressure, measured at 21 mm Hg during catheterization.

The subxiphoid examination (Figure 133) on the same patient whose tracing is seen in Figure 132 discloses a basilar left ventricular dimension within the normal limits. The septum does not appear to move well in the area of the mitral valve; the posterolateral wall continues to move normally. The apical dimension was somewhat dilated but not as grossly as that seen in Figure 132. Because the echogram suggested a large anterior apical ventricular aneurysm with well-preserved posterior and posterolateral wall motion and because of refractory congestive heart failure, cardiac catheterization was undertaken to ascertain if there was a potentially resectable ventricular aneurysm.

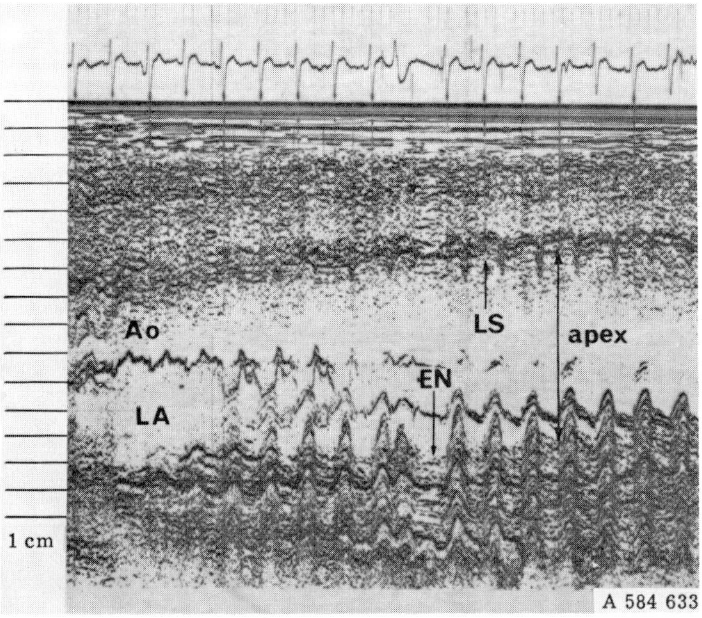

Figure 132. Male, age 72, admitted to hospital for regulation of insulin-dependent diabetes mellitus. Patient had history of arteriosclerotic heart disease with angina pectoris since 1960. The mid-to-low scan was recorded from left sternal border. Transducer is most perpendicular to septum and posterior wall slightly below mitral valve. Ao = aorta, LA = left atrium, LS = left septum and EN = endocardial surface of posterior left ventricular wall.

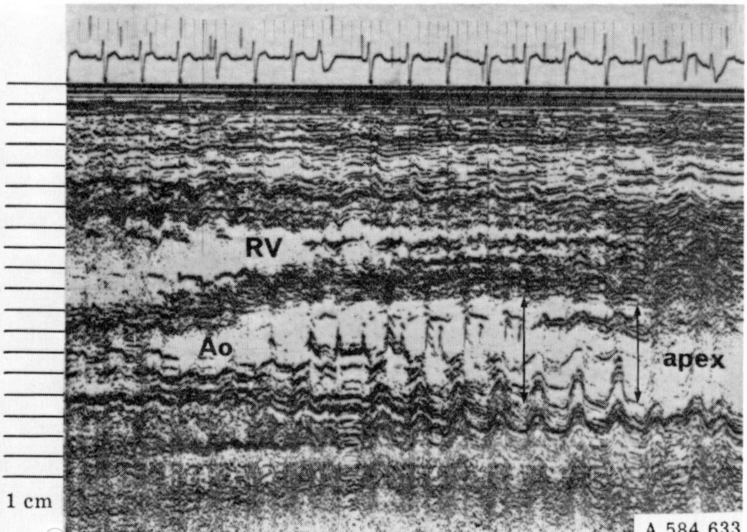

Figure 133. Subxiphoid condensed scan from same patient as in Figure 132. Basilar dimension is within normal limits; apex is slightly dilated. Septal motion is hypokinetic; posterolateral wall motion is normal. Disparity between left sternal border examination and subxiphoid examination is strongly suggestive of ventricular aneurysm. RV = right ventricle and Ao = aorta.

The surgeon's description of the left ventriculogram is: "The left ventricular cavity was markedly enlarged with marked generalized hypokinesis. Only small areas of the infero-basal and antero-basal portions of the left ventricle were contracting; the anterior apical, and inferior apical portions of the left ventricle were akinetic. The anterior basilar portion of the left ventricle was noted to have early relaxation. No discrete aneurysm was found."

It is interesting that the right anterior oblique cineangiogram gave an impression of diffuse hypokinesia; whereas the echogram identified areas of efficient muscular function, particularly the posterior and posterolateral portions of the left ventricle. A left anterior oblique angiogram was not done. The patient is being maintained on a medical regimen and is not considered to be a surgical candidate.

Because of the habitus of the coronary patient, tracings from multiple interspaces along the left sternal border are not always possible. The subxiphoid examination is usually successful, however. The patient whose tracings are depicted in Figures 134, 135 and 136 was one of the early subjects in whom multiple intercostal spaces and subxiphoid approach was used in an attempt to evaluate the left ventricle from several planes. By a comparison of the basilar and apical dimensions from these multiple planes and an analysis of the septal and posterior left ventricular wall motion, the diagnosis of ventricular

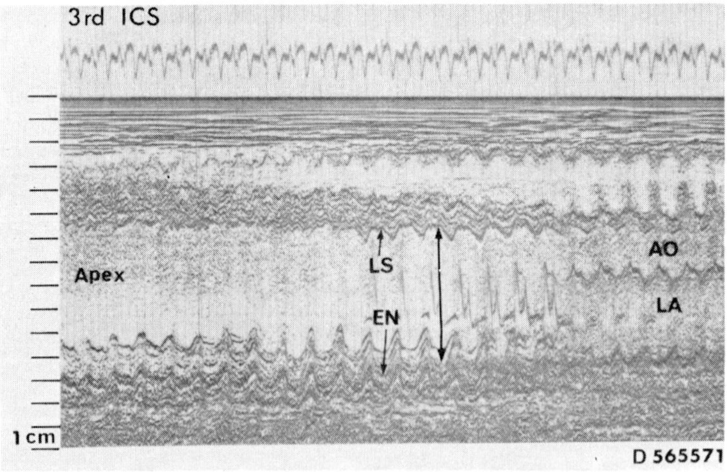

Figure 134. Condensed scan from third intercostal space along left sternal border. Basilar dimension is dilated, but anterior septal and posterior left ventricular wall motion is efficient. Wall motion toward apex appears to be diminished; this may be real or artifactual because sound beam is oblique to apical wall structures from this transducer position. LS = left septum, EN = endocardial surface of posterior left ventricular wall, AO = aorta and LA = left atrium.

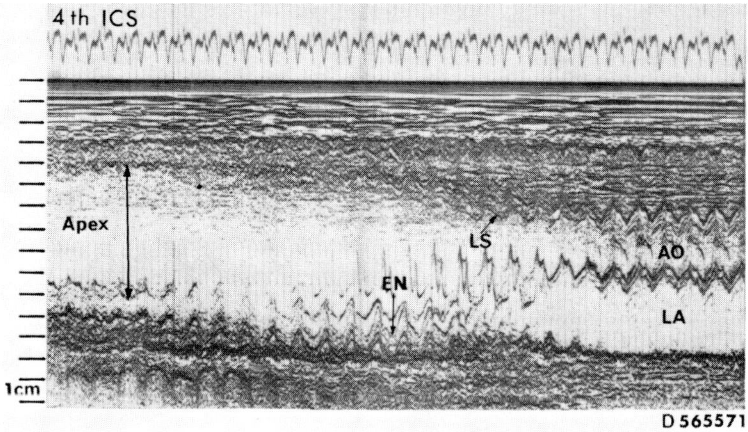

Figure 135. Condensed scan from fourth intercostal space of same 59-year-old patient as in Figure 134. Transducer has been positioned more laterally from left sternal border to place sound beam perpendicular to walls of apex. Scan from apex to aorta discloses dilated apex with akinetic septal motion. At operation there was an area approximately 12 cm long and 8 cm wide where muscle had been replaced by scar tissue. LS = left septum, EN = endocardial surface of posterior left ventricular wall, AO = aorta and LA = left atrium.

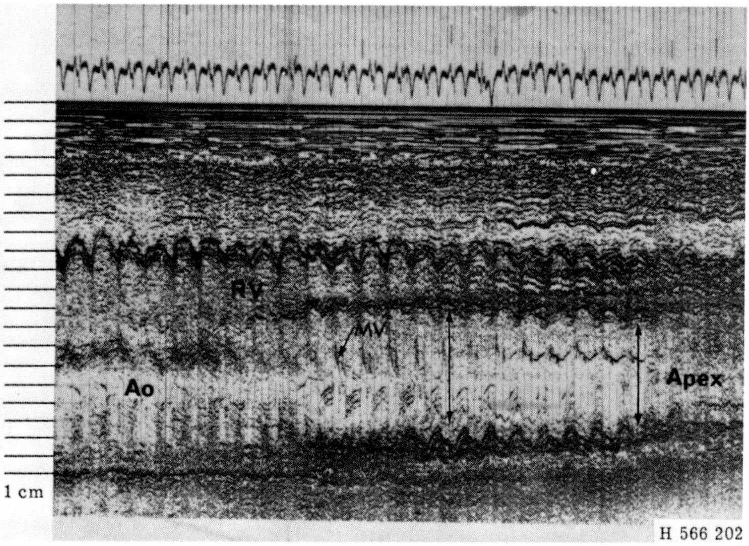

Figure 136. Subxiphoid scan from same patient whose tracings are depicted in Figures 134 and 135. Transducer was angled from tricuspid-aortic area to apex. Most remarkable features are efficient inferior septal wall motion and posterolateral wall motion from base to apex with effect of tapering evident as sound beam approaches apex. This tapering at apex is in sharp contrast to appearance of apex in Figure 135. Ao = aorta, RV = right ventricle and MV = mitral valve.

aneurysm was established. The patient subsequently underwent cardiac catheterization and surgical resection of the aneurysm.

The surgeon's description of the results of the right anterior oblique cineangiogram revealed: ". . . a moderate size dyskinetic segment in the anterolateral aspect of the left ventricle. Left coronary arteriograms revealed total occlusion of the mid left anterior descending artery. The remainder of the left coronary was unremarkable. The right coronary artery was also unremarkable."

Suggested Reading

Left Ventricle—General

Abbasi A., *et al.*: Ultrasound in the diagnosis of primary congestive cardiomyopathy. Chest *63*:937, 1973.

Bove, A., Ziskin, M., and Mulchin, W.: Ultrasonic detection of in vivo cavitation and pressure. Effects of high-speed injections through catheters. Invest. Radiol., *4*:236, 1969.

Chestler, E., Jaffe, H., and Vecht, R.: Ultrasound cardiography in single ventricle and hypoplastic left and right heart syndromes. Circulation *42*:123, 1970.

Chung, K., *et al.*: Echocardiographic findings in tetralogy of Fallot. Am. J. Cardiol., *31*:126, 1973.

Feigenbaum, H., *et al.*: Identification of ultrasound echoes from the left ventricle using intracardiac injections of Indocyanine Green. Circulation *41*:615, 1970.

Forker, A., Wilson, C., and Weaver, W.: Unexplained congestive heart failure: Value of echocardiography in detecting correctible disease. Nebr. Med. J., *59*:11, 1974.

Frishman, W., *et al.*: Heart failure 63 years after traumatic arteriovenous fistula. Am. J. Cardiol., *34*:733, 1974.

Frishman, W., *et al.*: Noninvasive assessment of clinical response to oral propranolol therapy. Am. J. Cardiol., *35*:635, 1974.

Gramiak, R., Shah, P., and Kramer, D.: Ultrasound cardiography: Contrast studies in anatomy and function. Radiology *92*:939, 1969.

Kerber, R., Kioschos, J., and Lauer, R.: Use of an ultrasonic contrast method in the diagnosis of valvular regurgitation and intracardiac shunts. Am. J. Cardiol., *34*:722, 1974.

King, D., Steeg, C., and Ellis, K.: Visualization of ventricular septal defects by cardiac ultrasonography. Circulation, *48*:1215, 1973.

Kones, R., and Phillips, J.: Foreign body of the heart complicated by papillary muscle necrosis located by echocardiography. Report of a case and review of the literature. Chest *62*:52, 1972.

Kronzon, I., *et al.*: Fixed membranous subaortic stenosis. Chest *67*:473, 1975.

McDonald, I., and Hobson, E.: A comparison of the relative value of noninvasive techniques—echocardiography, systolic time intervals and apexcardiography. Am. Heart J., *88*:454, 1974.

Murphy, K., *et al.*: Ultrasound in the diagnosis of congenital heart disease (review). Am. Heart J., *89*:638, 1975.

Oakley, C.: Clinical definitions and classifications of cardiomyopathies. Postgrad Med. J., *48*:703, 1972.

Schuilenburg, R., and Durrer, D.: Further observations on the ventricular echo phenomenon elicited in the human heart: Is the atrium part of the echo pathway? Circulation, *45*:629, 1972.

Smith, M., and Hood, W.: Echocardiographic patterns recorded from patient with a peripheral arterio-venous shunt. J. Clin. Ultrasound, *1*:288, 1973.

Tajik, A., *et al.*: Echocardiogram in Ebstein's anomaly with Wolff-Parkinson-White pre-excitation syndrome, Type B. Circulation, *47*:813, 1973.

Tajik, A., *et al.*: Echocardiogram in tetralogy of Fallot. Chest, *64*:107, 1973.

Yuste, P., *et al.*: Ultrasonics in the study of Ebstein's anomaly. Rev. Esp. Cardiol., *26*:339, 1973.

Left Ventricle—in IHSS

Abbasi, A., *et al.*: Echocardiographic diagnosis of idiopathic hypertrophic cardiomyopathy without outflow obstruction. Circulation, *46*:897, 1972.

Aigner, A., *et al.*: Asymmetric septal hypertrophy. Ann. Intern. Med., *81*:650, 1974.

Bloom, K., *et al.*: The association of fixed and dynamic left ventricular outflow obstruction. Am. Heart J., *89*:586, 1975.

Bolton, M., Jr., *et al.*: The effects of operation on the echocardiographic features of idiopathic hypertrophic subaortic stenosis. Circulation, *50*:897, 1974.

Chung, K., Manning, J., and Gramiak, R.: Echocardiography in coexisting hypertrophic subaortic stenosis and fixed left ventricular outflow obstruction. Circulation, *49*:673, 1974.

DeLaCalzada, C., *et al.*: Proceedings: Echocardiographic features of hypertrophic obstructive cardiomyopathy. Br. Heart J., *36*:396, 1974.

Hardarson, T., and Curiel, R.: Study of clinical pharmacology of hypertrophic obstructive cardiomyopathy by non-invasive diagnostic investigations. Br. Heart J., *35*:865, 1973.

Henry, W., Clark, C., and Epstein, S.: Asymmetric septal hypertrophy: The unifying link in the IHSS disease spectrum. Observations regarding its pathogenesis, pathophysiology and course. Circulation, *47*:827, 1973.

Henry, W., *et al.*: Echocardiographic measurement of the left ventricular outflow gradient in idiopathic hypertrophic subaortic stenosis. N. Engl. J. Med., *288*:19, 1973.

Johnson, A., Lonsky, S., and Carleton, R.: Combined hypertrophic subaortic stenosis and calcific aortic valvular stenosis. Am. J. Cardiol., *35*:706, 1975.

King, J., *et al.*: Markedly abnormal mitral valve motion without simultaneous interventricular pressure gradient due to uneven mitral-septal contact in idiopathic hypertrophic subaortic stenosis. Am. J. Cardiol., *34*:360, 1974.

King, J., *et al.*: Echocardiographic assessment of idiopathic hypertrophic subaortic stenosis. Chest, *64*:723, 1973.

Kossowsky, W., Mohr, B., and Dardashti, I.: Acute myocardial infarction in idiopathic hypertrophic subaortic stenosis. Chest, *64*:529, 1973.

Marcus, G., Popp, R., and Stinson, E.: Coronary-artery disease with IHSS. Lancet, *1*:901, 1974.

Nanda, N., *et al.*: Echocardiography in the diagnosis of idiopathic hypertrophic subaortic stenosis co-existing with aortic valve disease. Circulation, *50*:752, 1974.

Pridie, R., and Oakley, C.: Mechanism of mitral regurgitation in hypertrophic obstructive cardiomyopathy. Br. Heart J., *32*:203, 1970.

Rossen, R., *et al.*: Echocardiographic criteria in the diagnosis of idiopathic hypertrophic subaortic stenosis. Circulation, *50*:747, 1974.

Shah, P.: IHSS—HOCM—MSS—ASH? Circulation, *51*:577, 1975 (editorial).

Shah, P., *et al.*: Role of echocardiography in diagnostic and hemodynamic assessment of hypertrophic subaortic stenosis. Circulation, *44*:891, 1971.

Shah, P., *et al.*: Echocardiographic assessment of the effects of surgery and propranolol on the dynamics of outflow obstruction and hyperpranolol on the dynamics of outflow obstruction and hypertrophic subaortic stenosis. Circulation, *45*:516, 1972.

Tajik, A., and Giuliani, E.: Echocardiographic observations in idiopathic hypertrophic subaortic stenosis. Mayo Clin. Proc., *49*:89, 1974.

Left Ventricle—Performance

Belenkie, I., *et al.*: Assessment of left ventricular dimensions and function by echocardiography. Am. J. Cardiol., *31*:755, 1973.

Benzing, G., *et al.*: Evaluation of left ventricular performance: Circumferential fiber shortening and tension. Circulation, *49*:925, 1974.

Cooper, R., *et al.*: Ultrasound determinations of mean fiber-shortening rate in man. Am. J. Cardiol., *29*:257, 1972.

Cooper, R., *et al.*: Comparison of ultrasound and cineangiographic measurements of the mean rate of circumferential shortening in man. Circulation, *46*:914, 1972.

Danford, H., *et al.*: Echocardiographic evaluation of the hemodynamic effects of chronic aortic insufficiency with observations on left ventricular performance. Circulation, *48*:253, 1973.

Delgado, C., Fortuin, N., and Ross, R.: Acute effects of low doses of alcohol on left ventricular function measured by echocardiography. Circulation, *51*:535, 1975.
Feigenbaum, H.: Use of echocardiography to evaluate cardiac performance. *In* Cardiac Mechanics. Edited by I. Mirsky, D. N. Ghista, and H. Sandler. New York, John Wiley, pp. 203–231, 1974.
Follath, F., Schmitt, H., and Burkart, F.: Echocardiographic evaluation of left ventricular function. Schweiz. Med. Wochenschr., *103*:1776, 1973.
Fortuin, N., Hood, W., Jr., and Craige, E.: Evaluation of left ventricular function by echocardiography. Circulation, *46*:26, 1972.
Galbo, H., and Paulev, P.: Cardiac function during rest and supine cycling examined with a new noninvasive technique. J. Appl. Physiol., *36*:113, 1974.
Gibson, D.: Disordered left ventricular contraction associated with abnormalities of conduction: an echocardiographic study. Postgrad. Med. J., *48*:756, 1972.
Gibson, D., and Brown, D.: Assessment of disordered left ventricular contraction from simultaneous measurements of left ventricular pressure and dimension. Br. Heart J., *35*:862, 1973.
Gibson, D., and Brown, D.: Measurement of instantaneous left ventricular dimension and filling rate in man using echocardiography. Br. Heart J., *35*:1141, 1973.
Gibson, D., and Brown, D.: Use of echocardiography in the evaluation of left ventricular function. Proc. R. Soc. Med., *67*:140, 1974.
Gibson, D., and Brown, D.: Proceedings: Stress-strain characteristics of left ventricular myocardium in man. Br. Heart J., *36*:398, 1974.
Gibson, D., and Brown, D.: Relation between diastolic left ventricular wall stress and strain in man. Br. Heart J., *36*:1066, 1974.
Grossman, W., MacLaurin, L., and Stefadouros, M.: Left ventricular stiffness associated with chronic pressure and volume overloads in man. Circ. Res., *35*:793, 1974.
Grossman, W., *et al.*: Quantitative assessment of left ventricular diastolic stiffness in man. Circulation, *47*:567, 1973.
Horwitz, L., Atkins, J., and Leshin, S.: Role of the Frank-Starling mechanism in exercise. Circ. Res., *31*:868, 1972.
Karliner, J., *et al.*: Mean velocity of fiber shortening; a simplified measure of left ventricular myocardial contractility. Circulation, *44*:323, 1971.
Kraunz, R., and Kennedy, J.: Ultrasonic determination of left ventricular wall motion in normal man. Studies at rest and after exercise. Am. Heart J., *79*:36, 1970.
Kraunz, R., and Ryan, T.: Ultrasound measurements of ventricular wall motion following administration of vasoactive drugs. Am. J. Cardiol., *27*:464, 1971.
Layton, C., *et al.*: Assessment of left ventricular filling and compliance using an ultrasound technique. Br. Heart J., *35*:559, 1973.
Levitsky, S., and Merchani, F.: Non-invasive methods of measuring myocardial contractility. Surg. Annu., *5*:205, 1973.
Ludbrook, P., *et al.*: Posterior wall velocity: An unreliable index of total left ventricular performance in patients with coronary artery disease. Am. J. Cardiol., *33*:475, 1974.
Ludbrook, P., *et al.*: Comparison of ultrasound and cineangiographic measurements of left ventricular performance in patients with and without wall motion abnormalities. Br. Heart J., *35*:1026, 1973.
McDonald, I.: Assessment of myocardial function by echocardiography. Adv. Cardiol., *12*:221, 1974.
McDonald, I., Feigenbaum, H., and Chang, S.: Analysis of left ventricular wall motion by reflected ultrasound: Application to assessment of myocardial function. Circulation, *46*:14, 1972.
Murray, J., Johnston, W., and Reid, J.: Echocardiographic determination of left ventricular performance. Ann. Intern. Med., *72*:777, 1970.
Murray, J., Johnston, W., and Reid, J.: Echocardiographic determination of left ventricular dimensions, volumes and performance. Am. J. Cardiol., *30*:252, 1972.
Nimura, Y., Kunori, S., and Beppo, S.: UOG Ultrasoundcardiogram and left ventricular function. Jap. J. Clin. Med., *32*:297, 1974.
Orlando, E., *et al.*: Echocardiographic study of left ventricular function. G. Ital. Cardiol., *3*:414, 1973.
Orlando, E., *et al.*: Analysis of left ventricular wall motion by means of ultrasonics. G. Ital. Cardiol., *2*:234, 1972.

Paraskos, F., *et al.*: A noninvasive technique for the determination of circumferential fiber shortening in man. Circulation Res., *29*:610, 1971.
Pernod, J., *et al.*: Myocardial contraction. Study by ultrasonic echography (results in 200 normal patients). Nouv. Presse Med., *2*:2393, 1973.
Peterson, K., *et al.*: Comparison of isovolumic and ejection phase indices of myocardial performance in man. Circulation, *49*:1088, 1974.
Quinones, M., Gaasch, W., and Alexander, J.: Echocardiographic assessment of left ventricular function: With special reference to normalized velocities. Circulation, *50*:42, 1974.
Quinones, M., *et al.*: Echocardiographic determination of left ventricular stress-velocity relations in man: With reference to the effects of loading and contractility. Circulation, *51*:689, 1975.
Rankin, L., Moos, S., and Grossman, W.: Alterations in preload and ejection phase indices of left ventricular performance. Circulation, *51*:910, 1975.
Smithen, C., Wharton, D., and Sowton, E.: Independent effects of heart rate and exercise on left ventricular wall movement measured by reflected ultrasound. Am. J. Cardiol, *30*:43, 1972.
Stefadouros, M., *et al.*: Noninvasive study of effect of isometric exercise on left ventricular performance in normal man. Br. Heart J., *36*:988, 1974.
Weissler, A.: Noninvasive methods for assessing left ventricular performance in man. Am. J. Cardiol., *34*:111, 1974.
Wharton, C., Smithen, C., and Sowton, E.: Changes in left ventricular movement after acute myocardial infarction measured by reflected ultrasound. Br. Med. J., *4*:75, 1971.
Ziady, G., Hardarson, T., and Curiel, R.: The use of echocardiography to measure isometric contraction time. Am. Heart J., *89*:200, 1975.

Left Ventricle—Pericardial Effusion

Abbasi, A., Ellis, N., and Flynn, J.: Echocardiographic M-scan technique in the diagnosis of pericardial effusion. J. Clin. Ultrasound, *1*:300, 1973.
Abbasi, A., and Flynn, J.: The use of modified echocardiographic M-scan technique in the diagnosis of pericardial effusion. Proceedings of the Scientific Sessions of the American Institute of Ultrasound in Medicine, Philadelphia, October, 1972.
Ali-Regiaba, S., *et al.*: Treatment of uraemic pericarditis by anterior pericardiectomy. Lancet, *2*:12, 1974.
Anonymous: Ultrasound in the diagnosis of pericardial effusion. Chin. Med., *7*:411, 1973.
Arlien-Soborg, P., and Lomholt, P.: Echocardiographic demonstration of pericardial exudate. Ugeskr. Laeger, *134*:1289, 1972.
Bilek, J., Lukas, I., and Hula, J.: Echocardiography in pericardial effusion. Case report. Vnitr. Lek., *16*:428, 1970.
Cardello, P., McQuown, D., and Dollinger, M.: Ultrasound in diagnosis of parapericardial masses. JAMA, *227*:1124, 1974 (letter).
Casarella, W., and Schneider, B.: Pitfalls in the ultrasonic diagnosis of pericardial effusion. Am. J. Roentgenol., *110*:760, 1970.
Ellis, K., and King, D.: Pericarditis and pericardial effusion. Radiologic and echocardiographic diagnosis. Radiol. Clin. North Am., *11*:393, 1973.
Everett, E.: Pericarditis due to entamoeba histolytica. South Med. J., *65*:501, 1972.
Farooki, Z., Henry, J., and Green, E.: Hemophilus influenzae pericarditis associated with meningitis. Clin. Pediatr. (Phila.), *13*:609, 1974.
Feigenbaum, H.: Echocardiographic diagnosis of pericardial effusion. Am. J. Cardiol., *26*:475, 1970.
Follath, F., and Heierli, B.: Echocardiography in pericardial effusion. Schweiz. Med. Wochenschr., *104*(44):1572, 1974.
Gabor, G., Winsberg, F., and Bloom, H.: Electrical and mechanical alternation in pericardial effusion. Chest, *59*:341, 1971.
Glaser, J.: Echocardiographic diagnosis of septic pericarditis in infancy. J. Pediatr., *83*:697, 1973.
Goldberg, B., and Pollack, H.: Ultrasonically guided pericardiocentesis. Am. J. Cardiol., *31*:490, 1973.

Haider, R., *et al.*: Congenital pericardio-peritoneal communication with herniation of omentum into the pericardium. A rare cause of cardiomegaly. Br. Heart J., *35*:981, 1973.
Hamilton, C., and Christiansen, M.: Chronic pericardial effusion and autoimmune antibodies—a case report. Nebr. Med. J., *59*(9):351, 1974.
Horowitz, M., *et al.*: Sensitivity and specificity of echocardiographic diagnosis of pericardial effusion. Circulation, *50*:239, 1974.
Jaeger, M.: The pericardial effusions. Ther. Umsch., *30*:574, 1973.
Landry, M., Candardjis, G., and Queloz, J.: Echocardiographic diagnosis of pericardial effusion. Schweiz. Med. Wochenschr., *103*:1841, 1973.
Nomeir, A., *et al.*: Cardiac involvement in rheumatoid arthritis. Ann. Intern. Med., *79*:800, 1973.
Ratshin, R., Smith, M., and Hood, W., Jr.: Possible false-positive diagnosis of pericardial effusion by echocardiography in presence of large left atrium. Chest, *65*:112, 1974.
Rothman, L., *et al.*: Ultrasonic diagnosis of pericardial effusion. Circulation *35*:358, 1967.
Sakamoto, T., *et al.*: Unusual diastolic heart beat in pericardial effusion. Jap. Heart J., *13*:379, 1972.
Shabetai, R.: Cardiac tamponade and constrictive pericarditis diagnosis. I. J. Maine Med. Assoc., *63*:123, 1972.
Stein, L., Shubin, H., and Weil, M.: Recognition and management of pericardial tamponade. JAMA, *225*:503, 1973.
Werning, C.: Ultrasound diagnostics of pericardial effusion. Dtsch. Med. Wochenschr., *97*:816, 1972.
Wright, F.: The diagnosis of free and loculated pericardial effusions during haemodialysis by diagnostic radiology, isotope scintiscanning and ultrasound. Br. J. Clin. Pract., *26*:143, 1972.

Left Ventricle—Ventricular Wall Motion and Dimensions

Abbasi, A., *et al.*: Paradoxical motion of interventricular septum in LBBB. Circulation, *49*:423, 1974.
Assad-Morell, J., Tajik, A., and Giuliani, E.: Aneurysm of membranous interventricular septum: Echocardiographic features. Mayo Clin. Proc., *49*:164, 1974.
Assad-Morell, J., Tajik, A., and Giuliani, E.: Echocardiographic analysis of the ventricular septum. Prog. Cardiovasc. Dis., *17*:219, 1974.
Belenkie, I., *et al.*: Assessment of left ventricular dimensions and function by echocardiography. Am. J. Cardiol., *31*:755, 1973.
Burch, G., Giles, T., and Martinez, E.: Echocardiographic detection of abnormal motion of the interventricular septum in ischemic cardiomyopathy. Am. J. Med., *57*:293, 1974.
Burch, G., Giles, T., and Martinez, E.: Echocardiographic abnormalities of interventricular septum associated with absent Q syndrome. JAMA, *228*:1665, 1974.
Burggraf, G., and Craige, E.: Echocardiographic studies of left ventricular wall motion and dimensions after valvular heart surgery. Am. J. Cardiol., *35*:473, 1975.
Carson, P., and Kantes, L.: Left ventricular wall movement in heart failure. Br. Med. J., *4*:77, 1971.
Chang, S., and Feigenbaum, H.: Subxiphoid echocardiography. J. Clin. Ultrasound, *1*:14, 1973.
Chang, S., Feigenbaum, H., and Dillon, J.: Subxiphoid echocardiography: A review. Chest, *68*:233, 1975.
Chang, S., Feigenbaum, H., and Dillon, J.: Condensed M-mode echocardiographic scan of the symmetrical left ventricle. Chest, *68*:93, 1975.
Cope, G., *et al.*: Diastolic vibration of the interventricular septum in aortic insufficiency. Circulation, *51*:589, 1975.
Corya, B., *et al.*: Anterior left ventricular wall echoes in coronary artery disease; linear scanning with a single element transducer. Am. J. Cardiol., *34*:652, 1974.
Corya, B., *et al.*: Echocardiographic features of congestive cardiomyopathy compared with normal subjects and patients with coronary artery disease. Circulation, *49*:1153, 1974.

Diamond, M., *et al.*: Echocardiographic features of atrial septal defect. Circulation, *43*:129, 1971.
Dillon, J., Chang, S., and Feigenbaum, H.: Echocardiographic manifestations of left bundle branch block. Circulation, *49*:876, 1974.
Feigenbaum, H.: Echocardiographic examination of the left ventricle. Circulation, *51*:1, 1975 (editorial).
Feigenbaum, H., *et al.*: Ultrasound measurements of the left ventricle: A correlative study with angiography. Arch. Intern. Med., *129*:461, 1972.
Fogelman, A., *et al.*: Echocardiographic study of the abnormal motion of the posterior left ventricular wall during angina pectoris. Circulation, *46*:905, 1972.
Forker, A., Wilson, C., and Weaver, W.: Illustrative echocardiogram. Eisenmenger's syndrome, pulmonary valvular insufficiency and paradoxic septal motion. Chest, *65*:202, 1974.
Gibson, D.: Estimation of left ventricular size by echocardiography. Br. Heart J., *35*:128, 1973.
Goldstein, S., and Willem de Jong, J.: Changes in left ventricular wall dimension during regional myocardial ischemia. Am. J. Cardiol., *34*:56, 1974.
Gramiak, R., and Nanda, N.: Echocardiographic diagnosis of ostium primum septal defect. Circulation (Suppl. II), *45*:46, 1972.
Hagan, A., *et al.*: Ultrasound evaluation of systolic anterior septal motion in patients with and without right ventricular volume overload. Circulation, *50*:248, 1974.
Jacobs, J., *et al.*: Detection of left ventricular asynergy by echocardiography. Circulation, *48*:263, 1973.
Kerber, R., Dippel, W., and Abboud, F.: Abnormal motion of the interventricular septum in right ventricular volume overload. Experimental and clinical echocardiographic studies. Circulation, *48*:86, 1973.
King, D., Steeg, C., and Ellis, K.: Visualization of ventricular septal defects by cardiac ultrasonography. Circulation, *48*:1215, 1973.
Kraunz, R., and Kennedy, J.: Ultrasonic determination of left ventricular wall motion in normal man. Studies at rest and after exercise. Am. Heart J., *79*:36, 1970.
Kraunz, R., and Ryan, T.: Ultrasound measurements of ventricular wall motion following administration of vasoactive drugs. Am. J. Cardiol., *27*:464, 1971.
Kreamer, R., Kerber, R., and Abboud, F.: Ventricular aneurysm: Use of echocardiography. J. Clin. Ultrasound *1*:60, 1973.
McCann, W., Harbold, N., Jr., and Giuliani, E.: The echocardiogram in right ventricular volume overload. JAMA, *221*:1243, 1972.
McDonald, I.: Echocardiographic demonstration of abnormal motion of the interventricular septum in left bundle branch block. Circulation, *48*:272, 1973.
Manoli, S.: An intraventricular ultrasound method for measurement of left-ventricular dimensions. Biomed. Eng., *21*:333, 1974.
Morganroth, J., *et al.*: Comparative left ventricular dimensions in trained athletes. Ann. Intern. Med., *82*:521, 1975.
Petersen, J., *et al.*: Echocardiographic recognition of left ventricular aneurysm. Am. Heart J., *83*:244, 1972.
Popp, R., *et al.*: Effect of transducer placement on echocardiographic measurement of left ventricular dimensions. Am. J. Cardiol., *35*:537, 1975.
Sandler, H., and Alderman, E.: Determination of left ventricular size and shape. Circulation Res., *40*:1, 1974.
Sayaya, J., Longo, M., and Schlant, R.: Echocardiographic interventricular septal wall motion and thickness: A study in health and disease. Am. Heart J., *87*:681, 1974.
Seides, S., *et al.*: Echocardiographic findings in isolated, surgically created tricuspid insufficiency. Am. J. Cardiol., *35*:679, 1974.
Stefan, G., and Bing, R.: Echocardiographic findings in experimental myocardial infarction of the posterior left ventricular wall. Am. J. Cardiol., *30*:629, 1972.
Tajik, A., Gau, G., and Schattenberg, T.: Echocardiogram in atrial septal defect. Chest, *62*:213, 1972.
Tajik, A., Gau, G., and Schattenberg, T.: Echocardiogram in atrial septal defect with small left to right shunt. Chest, *63*:95, 1973.
Tajik, A., *et al.*: Normal ventricular septal motion in atrial septal defect. Mayo Clin. Proc., *47*:635, 1972.

Tallury, V., DePasquale, N., and Burch, G.: The echocardiogram in papillary muscle dysfunction. Am. Heart J., *83*:12, 1972.
Williams, R., and Rudd, M.: Echocardiographic features of endocardial cushion defects. Circulation, *49*:418, 1974.

Left Ventricle—Volumes

Branzi, A., *et al.*: Ultrasound determination of left ventricular position for volume angiography. Chest, *62*:29, 1972.
Burggraf, G., and Parker, J.: Left ventricular volume changes after amyl nitrite and nitroglycerin in man as measured by ultrasound. Circulation, *49*:136, 1974.
Fortuin, N., *et al.*: Determinations of left ventricular volumes by ultrasound. Circulation, *44*:575, 1971.
Kantrowitz, P., and Kingsley, B.: A survey of the clinical measurement of cardiac output. Med. Res. Eng., *10*:12, 1971.
MacKay, R.: Non-invasive cardiac output measurement. Microvasc. Res., *4*:438, 1972.
McLaurin, L., *et al.*: A new technique for the study of left ventricular pressure-volume relations in man. Circulation, *48*:56, 1973.
Pombo, J., *et al.*: Comparison of stroke volume and cardiac output determination by ultra sound and dye dilution in acute myocardial infarction. Am. J. Cardiol., *27*:630, 1971.
Pombo, J., Troy, B., and Russell, R., Jr.: Left ventricular volumes and ejection fraction by echocardiography. Circulation, *43*:480, 1971.
Popp, R., *et al.*: Ultrasonic cardiac echography for determining stroke volume and valvular regurgitation. Circulation, *41*:493, 1970.
Popp, R., *et al.*: Sources of error in calculation of left ventricular volumes by echography. Am. J. Cardiol., *31*:152, 1973.
Ratshin, R., *et al.*: Quantitative echocardiography: Correlations with ventricular volumes by angiography in patients with coronary artery disease with and without wall motion abnormalities. Circulation, *48* (Suppl.) IV:48, 1973.
Ratshin, R., Rackley, C., and Russell, R.: Serial evaluation of left ventricular volumes and posterior wall movement in the acute phase of myocardial infarction using diagnostic ultrasound. Am. J. Cardiol., *29*:286, 1972.
Ratshin, R., Rackley, C., and Russell, R.: Determination of left ventricular preload and afterload by quantitative echocardiography in man. Circ. Res., *34*:711, 1974.
Ratshin, R., *et al.*: The accuracy of ventricular volume analysis by quantitative echocardiography in patients with coronary artery disease with and without wall motion abnormalities. Am. J. Cardiol., *33*:164, 1974.
Redwood, D., Henry, W., and Epstein, S.: Evaluation of the ability of echocardiography to measure acute alterations in left ventricular volume. Circulation, *50*:901, 1974.
Stefadouros, *et al.*: The effect of isometric exercise on the left ventricular volume in normal man. Circulation, *49*:1185, 1974.
Suga, H., and Sagawa, K.: Assessment of absolute volume from diameter of the intact canine left ventricular cavity. J. Appl. Physiol., *36*:496, 1974.
TenCate, F., *et al.*: Dimensions and volumes of left atrium and ventricle determined by single beam echocardiography. Br. Heart J., *36*:737, 1974.

Left Ventricle—Wall Thickness

Abbasi, A., *et al.*: Left ventricular hypertrophy diagnosed by echocardiography. N. Engl. J. Med., *289*:118, 1973.
Askanas, A., Rajszys, R., and Sandowski, Z.: Measurement of the thickness of the left ventricular wall in man using the ultrasound technique. Pol. Med. J., *9*:62, 1970.
Bennett, D., and Evans, D.: Correlation of left ventricular mass determined by echocardiography with vectorcardiographic and electrocardiographic voltage measurements. Br. Heart J., *36*:981, 1974.
Grossman, W., *et al.*: Wall thickness and diastolic properties of the left ventricle. Circulation, *49*:129, 1974.
Sawaya, J., Longo, M., and Schlant, R.: Echocardiographic interventricular septal wall motion and thickness: A study in health and disease. Am. Heart J., *87*:681, 1974.
Sjögren, A., Hytonen, I., and Frick, M.: Ultrasonic measurements of left ventricular wall thickness. Chest, *57*:37, 1970.

Troy, B., Pombo, J., and Rackley, C.: Ultrasonic measurements of left ventricular wall thickness and mass. Circulation, *42* (III):38, 1970.
Troy, B., Pombo, J., and Rackley, C.: Measurement of left ventricular wall thickness and mass by echocardiography. Circulation, *45*:602, 1972.
Wirth, J., and Wenzelides, K.: Heart muscle thickening measurement with ultrasound. Cor Vasa, *12*:112, 1970.

Left Ventricle—Pediatric

Dillon, J.: Echocardiographic pattern of right ventricular diastolic volume overload in children. Circulation *47*:431, 1973.
Kaye, H., Tynan, M., and Hunter, S.: Validity of echocardiographic estimates of left ventricular size and performance in infants and children. Br. Heart J., *37*:371, 1975.
Lortscher, R., *et al.*: Echocardiographic determinations of dimensions of normal newborns at 5,280 feet elevation. J. Clin. Ultrasound, *2*:51, 1975.
Machida, K., *et al.*: Ultrasonic measurements of left ventricular volume, mass and velocity of posterior wall movement in children. Nippon Acta. Radiol., *33*:617, 1973.
Meyer, R., *et al.*: Ventricular septum in right ventricular volume overload: An echocardiographic study. Am. J. Cardiol., *30*:349, 1972.
Meyer, R., Stockert, J., and Kaplan, S.: Echocardiographic determination of left ventricular volumes in pediatric patients. Circulation, *51*:297, 1975.
Morganroth, J., *et al.*: Electrocardiographic evidence of left ventricular hypertrophy in otherwise normal children: Clarification by echocardiography. Am. J. Cardiol., *35*:278, 1975.
Sahn, D., *et al.*: Echocardiographic assessment of left ventricular performance in normal newborns. Circulation, *49*:232, 1974.
Tajik, A., *et al.*: Echocardiographic pattern of right ventricular diastolic volume overload in children. Circulation, *46*:36, 1972.

APPENDIX

Common Abbreviations

AAL = anterior aortic leaflet
AAW = anterior aortic wall
AI = aortic insufficiency
AMV = anterior mitral valve
AO, Ao = aorta
APV = anterior pulmonary valve
ARV = anterior right ventricular wall
AS = aortic stenosis
ASD = atrial septal defect
ASHD = atherosclerotic heart disease
ATV = anterior tricuspid valve
AV = aortic valve
C = catheter, close
CAD = coronary artery disease
Ca^{++} = calcium
Ch = chordae
CHF = congestive heart failure
cm = centimeter
COLD = chronic obstructive lung disease
EN = endocardium, endocardial surface of posterior left ventricular wall
Ep = epicardium
IHSS = idiopathic hypertrophic subaortic stenosis
IVS = interventricular septum
LA = left atrium
LS = left septum
LVID = left ventricular internal dimension
LVIDd = left ventricular internal dimension taken during diastole
LVIDs = left ventricular internal dimension taken during systole
LVOT = left ventricular outflow tract
M = mitral valve
mm = millimeter
MI = mitral insufficiency
MS = mitral stenosis
MV = mitral valve
O = open
P = prolapse, pericardium
PAL = posterior aortic leaflet
PAW = posterior aortic wall
PE = pericardial effusion

per, peri or peric	= pericardium	**RAL**	= right anterior aortic leaflet
PI	= pulmonary insufficiency	**RS**	= right septum
PLA	= posterior left atrial wall	**RVD**	= right ventricular dimension
PLV	= posterior left ventricular wall	**RVOT**	= right ventricular outflow tract
PMV	= posterior mitral valve	**S**	= sternum
PND	= paroxysmal nocturnal dyspnea	**sec**	= second
PPM	= posterior papillary muscle	**SOB**	= shortness of breath
PPV	= posterior pulmonary valve	**T**	= tumor, transducer
PS	= pulmonary stenosis	**TI**	= tricuspid insufficiency
PTV	= posterior tricuspid valve	**TRANS**	= transducer
PV	= pulmonary valve	**TS**	= tricuspid stenosis
PW	= posterior wall	**TV**	= tricuspid valve
		VCF	= velocity of circumferential fiber shortening
		Veg	= vegetations
		VSD	= ventricular septal defect

Reading A Routine Echogram

Rule: IF YOU CANNOT SEE IT, DO NOT ASSUME THE MOTION; NO INTERPRETATION IS BETTER THAN A WRONG ONE.

The tendency is to overread a tracing. There are some guidelines to follow when reading an echogram, but very often a judgment about every item *cannot* be made. It is not necessary to report on every aspect of the reading; only those items pertinent to making the diagnosis are useful in the echogram report. Additional items may be reported if individual patients are being followed serially.

RVD = right ventricular dimension

range:	supine	0.7–2.3 cm	ave = 1.5 cm
	left lateral	0.9–2.6 cm	ave = 1.7 cm

LVID = left ventricular internal dimension

range:	supine	3.7–5.6 cm	ave = 4.6 cm
	left lateral	3.5–5.7 cm	ave = 4.6 cm

LAD = left atrial dimension

range:	uncorrected	1.9–4.0 cm	ave = 2.9 cm
	corrected	1.2–2.2 cm/M^2	ave = 1.6 cm/M^2

Anterior septal wall thickness
range: 0.6–1.1 cm ave = 0.9 cm

Posterior left ventricular wall thickness
range: 0.6–1.1 cm ave = 0.9 cm

Anterior septal wall systolic amplitude
range: 0.4–0.8 cm ave = 0.5 cm

Inferior septal wall systolic amplitude
range: 0.5–1.2 cm ave = 0.7 cm

Posterior left ventricular wall systolic amplitude
range: 0.9–1.4 cm ave = 1.2 cm

Posterolateral left ventricular wall systolic amplitude
range: 0.9–1.4 cm ave = 1.0 cm

Systolic motion of anterior septum
Normal posterior displacement during systole:
0.4–0.8 cm amplitude, normal
<0.3 cm amplitude, reduced
>0.9 cm amplitude, exaggerated

Exaggerated septal motion may indicate aortic or mitral insufficiency, ventricular septal defect, patent ductus arteriosus, increased cardiac output, overcompensation for a dyskinetic, hypokinetic or akinetic segment of muscle elsewhere as in coronary artery disease.

Paradoxical anterior displacement of the septum with the onset of systole may indicate left bundle branch block (LBBB). If the right ventricular dimension is dilated, this septal motion may indicate atrial septal defect (ASD), pulmonic insufficiency (PI), tricuspid insufficiency (TI), anomalous pulmonary vein, pulmonary embolization or any combination of these; or technical problem owing to positioning of the heart within the chest cavity, *e.g.*, horizontally placed hearts.

Flattened septal motion (systolic amplitude <0.3 cm) may indicate possible left anterior descending (LAD) coronary artery obstruction or possible technical problem, usually solved by turning the patient to a more left lateral position or angling the transducer more laterally.

Motion of posterior left ventricular wall
Normal anterior displacement with onset of systole:
0.9–1.4 cm amplitude, normal
<0.8 cm, reduced
>1.5 cm, exaggerated

Reduced posterior wall motion may indicate myopathy, coronary artery disease, congestive failure, low cardiac output or technical problem of recording the full excursion of the wall.

Exaggerated posterior wall motion may indicate left ventricular volume overload or overcompensation for akinetic, dyskinetic or hypokinetic segments elsewhere as in coronary artery disease.

Paradoxical motion may indicate ventricular aneurysm or poor technique.

Motion of left atrial wall

$<$1.0 cm, normal
1.3 cm or $>$, exaggerated

Exaggerated left atrial wall motion may indicate increased left atrial stroke volume, as in mitral insufficiency (MI), or it may be nonspecific.

Mitral valve motion

Normal: cusps' separation, 2.6–3.7 cm
Reduced: cusps' separation, 2.5 cm and less
Increased: cusps' separation, 3.8 cm and greater

Are the cusps thickened? Look for subacute bacterial endocarditis, rheumatic heart disease or myxomatous degeneration.

Do the cusps separate in opposite directions with the onset of diastole? Look for normal mitral valve or mitral commissurotomy.

Does one cusp move normally but the other abnormally? Look for congenital mitral stenosis, mitral commissurotomy or ruptured posterior mitral leaflet.

Do both cusps move in the same direction? Look for mitral stenosis, left atrial tumor (posterior leaflet obscured by tumor) or calcification hiding true definition of posterior leaflet.

Is the atrial contraction to mitral closure time interval (PR–AC) prolonged? Look for elevated left ventricular end-diastolic pressure.

Does the mitral opening velocity appear slowed with an amputated "E" point and large atrial component? Look for elevated initial left ventricular diastolic pressure or aortic insufficiency.

Does the mitral valve bulge anteriorly during systole? Look for IHSS, pseudo-IHSS or mitral annulus.

Does the valve bulge posteriorly toward the left atrial wall during early or mid systole? Look for prolapsed mitral valve (both leaflets or only the posterior leaflet may prolapse; many variants; usually an overread).

Do the cusps flutter with fine vibrations? Look for aortic insufficiency, massive mitral insufficiency (rarely seen to flutter) or electronic vibrations.

Do the cusps flutter with coarse vibrations? Look for atrial fibrillation.

Is the space beneath the anterior cusp clear of organized echoes? Look for atrial myxoma (scan into the left atrium to be sure), calcification or SBE vegetations.

Aortic valve motion

Normal: cusps' separation, 1.5–2.6 cm

Are the cusps thin or thickened during either systole or diastole? If the cusps are thickened, this may indicate aortic insufficiency (leaflets do not coapt properly), aortic stenosis (leaflets thick and distorted from natural symmetry) or SBE vegetations.

Is one cusp thicker than the other? Is the movement of one cusp more than the other? This may indicate bicuspid aortic stenosis, sinus of Valsalva aneurysm or technical problem (examine questionable valves from many intercostal spaces).

Does the valve open initially and then tend to close in early systole? Depending on the degree of closure, this may indicate severe IHSS, discrete subaortic stenosis, small ventricular septal defect (unproven) or mitral insufficiency (unproven).

Does the valve open initially and then tend to drift toward a closed position? This may indicate low cardiac output attributable to congestive failure, myopathy or mitral insufficiency or stenosis.

Tricuspid valve motion

Does the valve flutter with fine vibrations? Look for pulmonary insufficiency.

Does the valve flutter with very coarse vibrations? Look for atrial fibrillation.

Is there prolonged A-C interval? Look for elevated right ventricular end-diastolic pressure.

Is the space beneath the cusp clear of organized echoes? Look for right atrial tumor, SBE or ruptured sinus of Valsalva aneurysm.

Is the closing velocity of the valve reduced? Look for tricuspid stenosis or a technical problem.

Pulmonary valve motion

Normal: maximum *a* wave depth during quiet inspiration 3–7 mm.

Mild pulmonary stenosis: *a* wave depth during quiet inspiration may be the same as normal.

Moderate pulmonary stenosis: maximum *a* wave depth during quiet inspiration is greater than 8 mm.

Severe pulmonary stenosis: valve is completely opened during atrial contraction and remains open prior to the onset of systole.

Infundibular pulmonary stenosis: valve exhibits gross vibrations with onset of systole and continues into early diastole.

Pulmonary hypertension: diastolic slope may be flat with absent *a* wave and midsystolic notching on the posterior leaflet.

Atrial fibrillation: no *a* wave.

Sinus rupture from aorta into right atrium: pulmonary valve opens prior to atrial contraction.

Adult Normal Values

	Range (cm)	*Mean (cm)*	*Number*
Age (years)	13 –54	26	134
BSA (M^2)	1.45– 2.22	1.8	130
RVD-flat	0.7 – 2.3	1.5	84
RVD-left lateral	0.9 – 2.6	1.7	83
LVID-flat	3.7 – 5.6	4.7	82
LVID-left lateral	3.5 – 5.7	4.7	81
Post. wall thickness	0.6 – 1.1	0.9	137
Post. LV wall amplitude	0.9 – 1.4	1.2	10
Post. lateral wall amplitude	0.9 – 1.4	1.2	38
Septal wall thickness	0.6 – 1.1	0.9	137
Ant. septal wall amplitude	0.3 – 0.8	0.5	10
Inf. septal wall amplitude	0.5 – 1.2	0.7	38
Left atrial dimension	1.9 – 4.0	2.9	133
Aortic root dimension	2.0 – 3.7	2.7	121
Aortic cusps' separation	1.5 – 2.6	1.9	93

Adult Normal Values, Corrected for Body Surface Area

RVD/M^2-flat	0.4 – 1.4	0.9	76
RVD/M^2-left lateral	0.4 – 1.4	0.9	79
LVID/M^2-flat	2.1 – 3.2	2.6	77
LVID/M^2-left lateral	1.9 – 3.2	2.6	81
LAD/M^2	1.2 – 2.2	1.6	127
Aortic root/M^2	1.2 – 2.2	1.5	115

Echocardiographic Consultation Form

The routine measurements on every patient are listed on sample echocardiographic consultation forms. Additional remarks should describe other abnormalities noted on the individual tracing. This additional information may include presence and approximate quantity of pericardial effusion. Description of the thickness; cusps' separation; velocity of opening; and pattern of diastolic closure of the mitral, aortic, tricuspid or pulmonary valves may be important in identifying valvular lesions. The amount of septal and posterior wall motion of the left ventricle may be important, especially in patients with coronary artery disease or volume overloads.

For those laboratories monitoring individual patients serially over a long interval, many more parameters may be desired and should be recorded on every consultation. The patient who is receiving medication that may alter the left ventricular function should probably have the velocity of circumferential fiber shortening (VCF) included as a part of the regular report. Patients with mitral stenosis, who are being monitored serially prior to a surgical procedure, should have the description of the valve thickness, presence of calcium and amplitude and velocity of closure included as a part of their regular consultation reports. Long-term postoperative monitoring of these patients would be done the same way.

We make no assumptions about the possible motion of any part of a tracing which is not plainly seen and recorded; seldom do we offer a specific diagnosis. We give generalizations that may point toward a possible diagnosis, such as right or left ventricular volume overload or probable coronary artery disease vs diffuse myocardial disease (unless both are severe; then we cannot tell the difference). Valvular disease lends itself to more specific diagnoses, such as moderate, calcific mitral stenosis or significant aortic insufficiency, or idiopathic hypertrophic subaortic stenosis vs prolapsing of the mitral valve.

The most important caveat to remember when reporting the results of an echogram is DON'T OVERREAD!

(Sample)

Echocardiographic consultation ______________________

Age___ Ht___ Wt___ Sex___ B.P.______

Inpatient ______ Outpatient______

Clinical impression and reason for examination:

____

__________________ M.D.
Requested by:

Interpretation:

	(cm)	Additional remarks
Right ventricular dimension	______	
Left ventricular dimension	______	
Left atrial dimension	______	
Posterior wall thickness	______	
Septal wall thickness	______	
Aortic root dimension	______	

Additional remarks:

Signature ______________________ M.D. __________________ Date

(Sample)

ECHOCARDIOGRAPHIC CONSULTATION

Name of Hospital ______________________ ______________________

Patient information: Age___ Ht____ Wt___

Preliminary diagnosis and reason for echogram:

____

____

______________________________________ ______________________ M.D.

Echo requested by

Interpretation:

	(cm)		
Right ventricular dimension	_____	Norm____	Dilat____
Left ventricular dimension (LSB)	_____	Norm____	Dilat____
Left ventricular dimension (subxiphoid)	_____	Norm____	Dilat____
Left atrial dimension	_____	Norm____	Dilat____
Aortic root dimension	_____	Norm____	Dilat____
Septal wall thickness	_____	Norm____	Dilat____
Posterior wall thickness	_____	Norm____	Dilat____

Pericardial effusion ______________________________________

Valvular motion: if abnormal, indicative of:

Mitral ______________________________________

Aortic ______________________________________

Tricuspid ______________________________________

Pulmonic ______________________________________

Additional remarks:

Signature ______________________________ M.D. Date __________

(sample)

Name of Hospital | Patient Information

ECHOCARDIOGRAM REPORT

ECHOCARDIOGRAPHIC DIMENSIONS

IN CENTIMETERS:

1. Right Ventricular Dimension: ________
2. Left Ventricular Dimension:
   A. End Diastolic: ________
   B. End Systolic: ________
3. Left Atrium: ________
4. Aortic Root: ________

IN MILLIMETERS:

5. Thickness of Left Ventricular Walls:
   A. Interventricular Septum: ________
   B. Posterior wall of the Left Ventricle: ________
6. Distance between the leaflets of Aortic Valve: ________
7. Slope of the anterior leaflet of the Mitral Valve: ________

DIAGNOSIS & REASON FOR ECHOCARDIOGRAM: ____________

____

DIAGNOSTIC FINDINGS:

____________________M.D.
Physician

(Sample)

Name of Hospital

Echocardiographic Consultation

Age____ Ht____ Wt____ M__ F__ Charge______

Inpatient ____ Outpatient____

Clinical impression and reason for examination:

____________ M.D.
Requested by

Interpretation:

Signature ______________________ M.D.__________________ Date

GLOSSARY

Amplitude of Motion

Amount of displacement of a structure from one point of reference to another. For example, the mitral valve opens from a closed position to an open position: the distance the mitral leaflet opens is the amplitude of that leaflet.

Bicuspid

The aortic valve in which two of the three cusps are fused together, the fused cusps being nearly immobile.

Bloom

A visual effect on a Polaroid film when the "clip" control is set too high. Two or more echoes that are very close fuse to form a wide, fuzzy echo.

Closing Velocity of Valve

The distance per second that a valve travels toward a closed position following completion of ventricular filling (diastole) or ventricular ejection (systole). The velocity of closure is expressed as mm/sec or cm/sec.

Crystal Artifact

The first signal (echo) seen anterior to the chest wall. If the coarse gain is set at low to moderate amplification and the near gain is turned completely off, the crystal artifact is the only echo remaining nearest to the transducer.

Eccentricity of Valve Opening

The diastolic position of the aortic valve within the confines of the anteroposterior aortic walls. The valve is eccentric if: 1.) the diastolic position of the aortic valve is too close to either aortic wall and 2.) the anterior or posterior cusp is nearly immobile; maximum valve opening would be accomplished by the more mobile leaflet.

Fibrosis

A thickening and toughening of tissue, usually descriptive of valvular tissue as in "fibrotic mitral stenosis"; may also describe area of ventricular muscle which has undergone scarring secondary to ischemic disease.

Gradient

Aortic, pressure difference between aorta and left ventricle during ventricular ejection (systole).
Mitral, pressure difference between left atrium and left ventricle during ventricular filling (diastole).
Tricuspid, pressure difference between right atrium and right ventricle during ventricular filling (diastole).
Pulmonary, pressure difference between right ventricle and main pulmonary artery during ventricular ejection (systole).

Homogeneous Material

Tissue of a similar density such as blood, ventricular muscle (myocardium), blood clot or pericardial effusion (fluid exudate between the epicardium and pericardium).

Interface

The point at which high-frequency sound leaves tissue of one density and enters another tissue of a different density. For example, the sound travels through blood and then ventricular muscle. The point at which the sound leaves the blood and enters the muscle is the "interface."

Lateral Beam Width

A transducer with a half-inch diameter transmits a sound beam which is a half-inch in diameter; by the time the beam reaches the posterior left ventricle, *e.g.*, it may be one inch in diameter. Some of the tissue falling within this one-inch diameter area will be reflected back to the transducer and seen on the oscilloscope with the original structural motion desired. Thus the examiner is able to see many structures that lie close together but not necessarily behind each other. Left ventricular endocardium, chordae of the mitral valve and trabeculations are seen and recorded simultaneously as structures in a linear relationship to each other, when in fact, some of these structures may be side by side, picked by the "lateral beam width."

Maximum Cusps Separation

The farthest distance two valvular leaflets separate from each other during diastole or systole.

MegaHertz (megacycle)

One megaHertz is an ultrasonic frequency equal to one million cycles per second.

Transducers are constructed to operate at frequencies of 1.0 megaHertz to 10.0 megaHertz. The most common frequency used for adult echocardiography is 2.25 megaHertz. This wavelength is forceful enough to penetrate to the most posterior aspects of cardiac tissue and define tissue interfaces which are roughly 1 mm apart.

M-Mode

Graphically recorded "motion" of a cardiac structure which constantly changes its location in reference to the transducer.

Multiple Echoes

More than one signal returned from a single structure. For example, the mitral valve is a curved structure that may reflect many signals from different points of curvature. These signals are visualized as multiple lines on the oscilloscope and on the paper record.

Peak of Atrial Contraction

The point at which the mitral or tricuspid valves have opened to their fullest extent following electrical atrial contraction, forcefully ejecting blood into the ventricles.

Resolution

The ability to visualize objects or interfaces that are very close together. If interfaces that lie 1 mm apart can be distinguished, this is considered excellent resolution in cardiac echography.

Sound Beam

The burst of high-frequency sound transmitted from the transducer every 1/1000 sec.

INDEX